Praise for The Secret Lives of Teeth

'Meliors Simms is now the leading authority on how our emotional and spiritual wellbeing affects our oral health. She writes with beautiful clarity, grace, compassion and wisdom. Her book is instantly accessible, well-researched, hugely informative, and full of helpful exercises to guide your own journey of health and understanding. Highly recommended.'
— *Dr Robin Youngson*
medical specialist, trauma therapist and author of Time to Care

'This insightful look into the connection between the mind and tooth archetypes is desperately needed for dentistry, to help mental health and overall wellbeing.'
— *Sonia Tai-Yo Pellerino*
biological Registered Dental Hygienist and founder of Nirvana Dental Apothecary

The Secret Lives of Teeth

Copyright © Meliors Simms 2023

First published 2023 by Holistic Tooth Fairy Limited,
Raglan, Aotearoa New Zealand
www.holistictoothfairy.com

All rights reserved

No part of this book may be reproduced or transmitted in any form or by any means, electronic or mechanical, including photocopying, recording or by any information storage and retrieval system, without prior permission in writing from the publisher.

A catalogue record for this book is available from the National Library of New Zealand.

Soft cover ISBN 978-1-9911927-0-7

This publication is designed to provide educational information about the subject matter covered. It is sold with the understanding that neither the author nor the publisher is engaged in rendering dental, medical, psychological or other professional services. While the publisher and author have used their best efforts in preparing this book, they make no representations or warranties with respect to the accuracy or completeness of the contents of this book. The advice and strategies contained herein may not be suitable for your situation. You should consult with a professional when appropriate.

Book cover illustration and internal illustrations by Meliors Simms

Design & layout www.yourbooks.co.nz

The Secret Lives of Teeth

UNDERSTANDING EMOTIONAL INFLUENCES ON ORAL HEALTH

MELIORS SIMMS

Dedicated to
my beloved father, Dr Norman Simms (1940–2022)
and to my coaching clients who went deep

TABLE OF CONTENTS

Disclaimer 1

Part I: A Guidebook 3
Introduction 5
1. Root Cause 13
2. A Cabinet of Curiosities 24
3. A Manifesto for Metaphysical Healing 36

Part II: An Atlas 49
4. Mapping the Landscape of Your Mouth 51
5. Mapping with Mouth Meridians 58
6. Mapping Quadrants of the Mouth 64
7. Mapping Types of Teeth 68
8. Mapping Tooth Surfaces 81

9. Mapping with Tooth Archetypes 84
    Nurturer archetype: Upper left central incisor (9) 85
    Leader archetype: Upper right central incisor (8) 86
    Beast archetype: Lower right central incisor (25) 87
    Doll archetype: Lower left central incisor (24) 88
    Priestess archetype: Upper left lateral incisor (10) 90
    Inner Critic archetype: Upper right lateral incisor (7) ... 91
    Guardian archetype: Lower right lateral incisor (26) 92
    Martyr archetype: Lower left lateral incisor (23) 93
    Submission archetype: Upper left canine (11) 95
    Commander archetype: Upper right canine (6) 96
    Collaborator archetype: Lower right canine (27) 97
    Servant archetype: Lower left canine (22) 98
    Forgiveness archetype: Upper left first premolar (12) .. 100
    Daddy archetype: Upper first premolar (5) 101
    Friend archetype: Lower right first premolar (28) 102
    Lover archetype: Lower left first premolar (21) 103
    Harvest archetype: Upper left second premolar (13) ... 104
    Alliance archetype: Upper right second premolar (4) .. 105
    Trust archetype: Lower left second premolar (20) 106
    Rival archetype: Lower left second premolar (29) 107
    Earth Mother archetype: Upper left first molar (14) ... 108
    Sun archetype: Upper right first molar (3) 109
    Professional archetype: Lower right first molar (30) ... 111
    Home archetype: Lower left first molar (19) 112
    Night archetype: Upper left second molar (15) 113
    Name archetype: Upper right second molar (2) 114
    Goals archetype: Lower right second molar (31) 115

    Conception archetype: Lower left second molar (18) .. 116
    Virtues archetype: Upper left wisdom tooth (16) 117
    Lore archetype: Upper right wisdom tooth (1) 118
    Mystic archetype: Lower right wisdom tooth (32) 120
    Honor archetype: Lower left wisdom tooth (17) 121
10. Symptoms as Messengers.. 122
    Abscesses and infections 125
    Ankylosed tooth 126
    Bruxism, jaw clenching and TMJD 127
    Canker sores 130
    Cracking, chipping or breaking teeth 130
    Decay.. 132
    Gum conditions... 133
    Missing teeth 137
    Retained baby teeth 139
    Root problems 140
    Plaque and tartar 142
    Sensitive teeth 143

Part III: A Toolkit... 145
11. Treasury of Transformative Tools............................... 147
12. Healing with Grace... 171

Appendix of Journaling Prompts..................................... 176
References 182
Index.. 186
Acknowledgements 194
About the author.. 196

DISCLAIMER

This book is about the metaphysical – non-physical – influences on your oral health, but it's important to also provide all the necessary physical support for your teeth and gums. Energetic and emotional approaches complement, but should not replace, mindful oral hygiene, appropriate dental care and healthy eating.

When choosing to act on information provided in this book, you need to consider your other health issues, and do your own research to confirm whether your actions are appropriate for you. You need to take responsibility for your own health and well-being.

Metaphysical approaches to oral health are not a substitute for seeing a dentist, dental hygienist or a doctor. If your teeth and gum health deteriorate or pain persists, you should seek advice from a dentist or a doctor.

I am not a dental practitioner and I am not offering any kind of medical or dental advice. I try to provide valuable information, but I cannot be responsible for the use that you make of that information.

The suggested activities and other recommendations made in this book are for educational and informational purposes only, to help you make better health decisions in conjunction with your regular treating practitioners. In choosing to follow any of these suggestions, you are taking responsibility for your own actions. Please use common sense and make independent inquiries before deciding to apply the information here to your circumstances.

Content warning

Some parts of this book mention sexual abuse and other traumatic experiences including dental misadventures.

Part I: A Guidebook

I acknowledge that the roots of my theory and practice are indebted to traditional and indigenous knowledge from many parts of the world. My approach to natural oral health stands on the shoulders of ancestors as I learn and relearn these concepts. I pay my deepest respects and give heartfelt thanks to traditional knowledge keepers past and present.

Meliors Simms

INTRODUCTION

Welcome to your mouth and its secrets, hidden within the familiar landscape of your teeth and gums. Your mouth, the site of so many mundane (and pleasurable) activities, can often also be a source of anxiety or shame.

Measured against the glossy veneered smiles you see on screens, your teeth can seem disordered: perhaps crowded, discolored or missing, sometimes weak, sensitive or painful. Unlike the photoshopped arches of perfect pink gums in toothpaste ads, your gums may seem to be in sad retreat or spitefully bleeding from a touch of floss.

You hear people talk about having 'good teeth' or 'bad teeth' as though teeth represent one's virtuous compliance with social expectations. Heroines flash blinding grins while villains grimace around rotten, crooked pegs. In capitalist societies, only poor adults have missing teeth because for enough money, or the right insurance, dentists can repair or replace almost any dental problem. A glance in your mouth as you speak can instantly lead anyone to make assumptions about your economic status, geographic mobility, or physical vulnerability.

In this book, all teeth are considered good teeth, no matter how much grief they've caused. Troublesome teeth or gums are only calling for you to pay attention to issues perceived as threatening to your body, psyche or soul, whether past or present.

Dear reader, I'm addressing this book to *you* directly as though, like me, you have worried about your own teeth at some point in your life. Whenever I see anyone with teeth or gum troubles, I feel much tenderness, compassion and empathy, and mostly it's you I've pictured in my mind as I've written the following pages.

I expect that many readers have picked up this book out of curiosity that there could be more to dental problems than floss and sugar. I also invite readers who are blessed with resilient teeth and gums to learn about the role your mouth might play in speaking soul truths.

This book has much to offer complementary health practitioners, therapists and coaches whose clients want to understand more about their teeth or gum issues. Kinesiologists and energy healers may return frequently to these pages in your work.

I respectfully salute dental professionals interested in extending the scope of advice you offer your patients. This book can help to open deeper conversations when your patients ask *why* they have symptoms, and to empower them to engage more collaboratively in their oral health.

Whatever your reason for reading, I hope you will approach this book with both an open mind *and* a healthy dose of skepticism. Ask yourself, does this ring true for me? Does it make sense with what I know to be true?

You may be tempted to jump to the middle chapters to look up the meaning of a particular tooth or the interpretation of a certain symptom before closing the covers and walking away. For some readers, this approach could provide just enough information to expand your own therapeutic practice to help improve your oral health.

However, this book is intended to work like a guidebook, rather than a dictionary. Here, you can access the grammar and culture of your teeth and gums, not just reference a new vocabulary. If you really want to enable sustained healing and transform your relationship with your teeth and gums, it's vital to understand and respond to your mouth's specific, personal messages about your unique circumstances. Reading all of this book will help you to hold deep and meaningful conversations with your mouth, which could lead to a wonderful lifelong friendship.

WHAT TO EXPECT

The Secret Lives of Teeth is the first in a series, each of which will focus on a different aspect of oral health. The book you are reading now offers a comprehensive overview of metaphysical influences on teeth and gums.

Book Two, *The Empowered Dental Patient* (2024), will cover tactics for overcoming dental anxiety, factors to consider when making dental decisions as well as protocols and practices to help ensure the best outcome from any dental experience. Book Three will provide a comprehensive introduction to effective physical self-help strategies for preventing and healing dental problems and maintaining strong healthy teeth and gums; including nutrition, hygiene, herbs, oral posture, jaw relaxation, as well as home remedies to relieve toothache and infection, remineralize cavities and decay, balance the oral microbiome, stabilize receding gums and more.

Here's an overview of what to expect in this first book, *The Secret Lives of Teeth*.

PART I: A GUIDEBOOK

Chapter 1: Root Cause provides context to explain how oral health can embody your emotional experiences as a member of your family, community and society. This chapter tells the story of my personal dental troubles, and how I learned how to use holistic strategies to save my remaining teeth.

Chapter 2: Cabinet of Curiosities offers a new perspective on the familiar anatomy, biology and physiology of your mouth. Understand how stress, trauma and emotional patterns can affect oral health and well-being through a lens of recent neurobiological research. The concepts, language and imagery of your mouth's physiological features can become a powerful metaphysical tool for healing the physical body.

Chapter 3: A Manifesto for Metaphysical Healing is offered as guard rails to help keep you safe as you apply metaphysical theories to individual experiences. The principles provide practical advice to follow as you read the following chapters.

PART II: AN ATLAS

Chapter 4: Mapping the Landscape of Your Mouth unpacks the difference between two categories of metaphysical theory which can be combined to build layers of emotional and psychological correspondences onto specific parts of your mouth. This chapter introduces the existing literature of metaphysical theories of oral health.

Chapter 5: Mapping with Mouth Meridians explains the meridian system of traditional Chinese medicine and how it connects each part of the mouth with the rest of the body via energy channels governed by different emotions.

Chapter 6: Mapping Quadrants of the Mouth describes the themes associated with the top, bottom, left, right, front and back of the mouth and is most useful for anyone dealing with symptoms that are localized in just one section of the mouth.

Chapter 7: Mapping Types of Teeth provides interpretations for symptoms which show up on a particular type of tooth i.e. incisors, canines, premolars, molars or wisdom teeth. These psychosocial associations are drawn largely from the work of Dr Michèle Caffin.

Chapter 8: Mapping Tooth Surfaces summarizes a perspective which applies a unique meaning to each individual surface or plane of each tooth offered by Dr Christian Beyer's 'dental decoding' theories.

Chapter 9: Mapping with Tooth Archetypes introduces the framework I have developed, Tooth Archetypes, in which each of the thirty-two adult teeth are described with detailed character studies drawn from my coaching experiences with hundreds of people all over the world.

Chapter 10: Symptoms as Messengers is a directory of the metaphysical associations for diseases, imbalances and injuries specific to the mouth, including abscesses and infections, an ankylosed tooth, bruxism, bite and TMJ, canker sores or aphthous ulcers, cracking, chipping or breaking teeth, decay (caries and cavities), gum conditions (gingivitis, periodontitis, receding gums, gum pockets and bone loss), missing teeth, retained baby teeth, root problems (nerve damage, non-vital tooth or resorption), plaque and tartar, and sensitive teeth.

PART III: A TOOLKIT

Chapter 11: A Treasury of Transformational Tools brings the theories home, with practical exercises to help you apply personal insights, and enable healing. Making sense of your oral issues can be like putting together a jigsaw puzzle where the picture is mostly blue sky. This chapter provides suggestions to invite transformation with relaxed curiosity and a playful spirit.

Chapter 12: Healing with Grace summarizes this book's robust, flexible, pragmatic approach to metaphysical oral health. Symptoms are your system's attempt to bring you into balance, which requires delicacy, nuance, and consistent practice in your unique circumstances.

An Appendix of Journaling Prompts provides suggestions for writing exercises to enhance the healing potential of your insights from this book.

The Secret Lives of Teeth is based on the premise that there can be emotional, energetic, spiritual, ancestral and psychological influences on the development of cavities, gum recession and other symptoms of oral ill health. With a narrow but deep focus on the emotional, psychological, spiritual and collective influences on your teeth and gums, I invite you to explore a new, complementary way to explore the question of 'why?'

NOTES ON NAMING AND NUMBERING TEETH

In order to work with Tooth Archetypes and tooth type associations, you'll need to know which individual tooth, or type of tooth, you are interpreting. If you aren't sure which is which, ask your dentist to share a copy of your dental chart. Most dental charts use one of three major numbering systems common to different parts of the world.

This book uses the Universal numbering system, which is most common in the United States of America. The World Health Organization's FDI (ISO 3950) system is used internationally. Palmer notation is an older system still used by most dentists in the United Kingdom.

The common names and Universal numbers used in this book

INTRODUCTION

are shown in bold in the table below. Unless otherwise indicated, all teeth referred to in this book are adult or permanent teeth, not baby, milk or deciduous teeth.

Tooth Type	Position	Universal	FDI	Palmer
Wisdom, third molar	Upper right back	1	18	8
Second molar	Upper right back	2	17	7
First molar	Upper right side	3	16	6
Second premolar, second bicuspid	Upper right side	4	15	5
First premolar. First bicuspid	Upper right side	5	14	4
Canine, cuspid, eye tooth	Upper right front	6	13	3
Lateral incisor	Upper right front	7	12	2
Central incisor	Upper right front	8	11	1
Central incisor	Upper left front	9	21	1
Lateral incisor	Upper left front	10	22	2
Canine, cuspid, eye tooth	Upper left front	11	23	3
First premolar, first bicuspid	Upper left side	12	24	4
Second premolar, second bicuspid	Upper left side	13	25	5
First molar	Upper left side	14	26	6
Second molar	Upper left back	15	27	7
Wisdom, third molar	Upper left back	16	28	8
Wisdom, third molar	Lower left back	17	38	8
Second molar	Lower left back	18	37	7

Tooth Type	Position	Universal	FDI	Palmer
First molar	Lower left side	19	36	6
Second premolar, second bicuspid	Lower left side	20	35	5
First premolar, first bicuspid	Lower left side	21	34	4
Canine, cuspid	Lower left front	22	33	3
Lateral incisor	Lower left front	23	32	2
Central incisor	Lower left front	24	31	1
Central incisor	Lower right front	25	41	1
Lateral incisor	Lower right front	26	42	2
Canine, cuspid,	Lower right front	27	43	3
First premolar, first bicuspid	Lower right side	28	44	4
Second premolar, second bicuspid	Lower right side	29	45	5
First molar	Lower right side	30	46	6
Second molar	Lower right back	31	47	7
Wisdom, third molar	Lower right back	32	48	8

Table of numbers and names for teeth

1.

ROOT CAUSE

At 3 am the tooth called Rival was throbbing like a siren, intense but diffuse, pounding the front of my head from the inside, but not yet recognizable as a toothache.

My pain slid from ten out of ten down to a nine when I hauled myself up on a bank of pillows. I stumbled to the bathroom for pills, which eventually dulled the pain to a mere six.

Through a thudding fog of agony and exhaustion, I tried to calm my breathing and anxious thoughts. Then I remembered feeling this exact kind of pain before, and the outcome it led to every other time.

Tears started to leak as I pleaded with my body, 'not another root canal'. There was nothing untoward noted in my last dental check-up just a few months earlier, but all my other root canals also came crashing in without warning.

More clarity came with the early morning light, but no peace. The pain started to concentrate into my lower right jaw, confirming its dental origins. At 8 am I started calling around to find a dentist who could see me straight away.

Every one of my six root canals started this way. They also each occurred in, or soon after, a rootless period of my life involving homelessness, immigration or extended travel. However, it was only much later that I saw the overlap between my tooth roots clamoring for attention and my nervous system's inherited preference for flight over fight.

When I was seventeen, an ancestral and personal pattern of running away from trouble served to weaken the energetic roots of an upper incisor bearing the Inner Critic archetype. I had my first root canal after leaving my hometown to escape from anti-Semitic bullying and crushing depression. While hitchhiking and couch surfing, a mysterious onslaught of horrific pain was only relieved by a humiliating dental school root canal procedure.

The experience was a wakeup call to embrace more vigilant oral hygiene and regular dental visits. Nonetheless, almost every check-up for the next three decades resulted in more fillings and every few years another root canal, crown or extraction. Dental interventions usually brought me some respite from pain but did nothing to relieve the feelings of shame, disappointment and frustration about the state of my teeth.

Through all those years I was consistent with my brushing and flossing habits, conscientious about healthy eating and mostly compliant with the advice I received at my frequent dental check-ups. Yet nothing I did ever seemed to stop the decline. I couldn't understand why there wasn't a correlation between my oral health habits and their results. Dentists subtly, or not so subtly, blamed my supposed bad habits, but I felt that was unjust because I conscientiously followed their advice.

Like most people, I was taught that any problems with my teeth proved I'd failed to comply with the three commandments of mainstream oral health advice, first learned from parents and

teachers, absorbed through media and marketing, and reinforced by dentists:
1. *Brush and floss daily.*
2. *Avoid sugary drinks and food.*
3. *Get regular dental check-ups and cleanings.*

In my late twenties, the roots of a left molar carrying the Home archetype were compromised after three years of international travel as a single mother. I was prescribed a root canal for unbearable yet unfocused jaw pain when I landed back in my parents' house almost 15 years after leaving. Unfortunately, the dentist mistakenly removed the healthy nerve of the adjacent molar (Conception archetype) leaving me in pain for another week before I went back to have the procedure repeated.

Within six months both of those root canals failed and had to be redone by another dentist. A couple of years later they failed again so I chose to have them extracted rather than go through another expensive attempt to save the teeth. Each surgery felt like a failure, not just of my body but also of the dental profession.

Underlying influences

Under the harsh lights of a dental clinic, considering emotional, energetic, ancestral, relational and collective influences on oral health may seem ridiculous, even primitive. Like the rest of Western medicine, dentistry has always considered mind and body as separate. Dentists almost always treat their patients' mouths with little reference to the rest of their body, let alone their thoughts and feelings. Mainstream dentistry tends to address oral health in isolation, as an individual responsibility and an individual virtue.

However, my chronic dental troubles came to an end only when I learned that sometimes, for some people, the basic tenets of oral health and dental care aren't enough; that even when you attend to those immediate physical needs, your mouth may continue to present problems. I started to understand that my oral health required a systemic, whole human approach that contextualizes teeth and gums in a web of relationships and environments, both past and present.

The first turning point for my teeth was finding out about the influence of nutrition; not just which foods to avoid, but what nutrients your teeth need to be healthy. Furthermore, teeth and gums interact with complex internal systems that are influenced by your whole physical body, including your posture, your breathing and your gut, what you inhale as well as what you eat and drink, your oral hygiene products and habits.

There are also external influences which can have a more delayed impact on teeth including genetics, prenatal, infant or childhood exposure to drugs or environmental toxins, parasites, malnutrition, disordered eating or mouth piercings, not to mention violent causes of immediate harm to oral health including accidental injuries or dental misadventure.

Yet, I always knew that there's more to me than my physical body. Humans are also made up of thoughts and emotions; we have psyche, soul and spirit. Like all beings, humans have a life force also known as energy, qi, prana, or mauri, which can be experienced as physical sensations and interpreted through thoughts and emotions, but which is itself ineffable (unable to be explained).

Your oral health is influenced by metaphysical factors such as your emotional state now, and in the past, including:

*Your family history, your ancestors' traumas,
and perhaps even past lives.
Your parents' circumstances and emotions
during your gestation, infancy and childhood.
Your adverse childhood experiences,
trauma or attachment-based hurts.*

Your attitudes and your beliefs.
Where you live, when you've moved, and how you travel.
Your stress levels, your hopes and your aspirations.
What you do every day, the people who talk to you
and the people you live with.
What you're angry about and what frustrates you.
Your disappointment and grief, your fear and anxiety.
The secrets that you keep, what you put up with, and
what you don't do or say.

Metaphysical influences can make you more vulnerable to physical threats. Physical influences can exacerbate metaphysical factors. The exact combination and timing of the underlying reasons for your teeth and gum issues are unique to you. Understanding the stories behind your symptoms can be just as important for your oral health as any dental or home remedy that you can use.

WHY ME, WHY NOW?

This book describes systems of metaphysical thought based on ideas about qi, emotional patterns, neurological development and social context in relation to oral health. Here you can read summaries of the most robust theories that I've teased out from scattered and patchy sources. I've tested these theories against my personal experience and used them in my coaching. The information in this book has helped hundreds of my clients to effectively address a wide variety of teeth and gum issues (both with, and without, dental interventions).

As a natural oral health coach, I meet (in video calls) with people of all ages, genders, races and cultures from all over the world, with varying levels of English fluency and diverse cultural references (although many are holistic healers in various modalities). Their diversity gave me a robust laboratory to test and refine a sensitive metaphysical toolkit, which is described in Chapter 11.

Out of necessity, I adapted existing esoteric theories into relatable language and imagery to help my clients understand why *that* symptom showed up in *that* part of their mouth at *that* time. Weaving together a review of the existing approaches to metaphysical oral health with my own Tooth Archetypes framework makes this the most comprehensive book about the metaphysics of oral health to be published in the English language to date.

Readers may be surprised to discover new ways to explore questions that aren't always satisfactorily explained by your dentist such as:

- *Why are some people's mouths prone to problems despite regular dental visits, conscientious oral hygiene and minimal sugar, but other people have impeccable oral health despite their lackadaisical habits?*
- *Why do some of your teeth get decay, even though you brush regularly, while other teeth stay strong and healthy?*
- *Why do gums recede around some teeth, even when you floss carefully, while other areas of gum hold tight to their teeth?*
- *And most of all, why does disease and decay in the mouth sometimes get worse, sometimes get better or sometimes linger at a low level over the long term, regardless of dental or self-help interventions?*

When you consider symptoms as more than physical phenomena, their apparent unpredictability starts to make more sense. Teeth are asking for attention when they present you with discomfort or decay. Your gums have something to say when they bleed or recede. Your mouth is attempting to communicate the need to change something in your life that's having a direct effect on your well-being.

RELATIONAL AND COLLECTIVE INFLUENCES

When your feelings have been suppressed instead of expressed, internalized emotions become embodied in the cells of your mouth, even influencing DNA to be passed down through families and affecting the oral health of later generations. Teeth can store the energetic memories of trauma, which may be from your own lifetime; inherited from your ancestors' experiences; or absorbed as collective memories from wars, natural disasters, pandemics, slavery and other wide-scale events.

Trauma may affect your teeth or gums through your personal experiences (primary trauma), or by witnessing someone else's trauma or acting as a perpetrator of trauma (secondary trauma). Primary and secondary traumas can compound and activate each other. Both types of individual trauma are underpinned by historical, collective, intergenerational, ancestral or institutionalized traumas such as racism, sexism, homophobia etc. (Menakem).

When you are not able to release or integrate emotions at the time of a traumatic event or soon after, the energetic residue of the trauma can get stored in your body. When a traumatic experience or its aftermath involves an imperative to be silent, the mouth may become the body part most likely to carry its residue.

Later, stress or post-traumatic stress disorder (PTSD) triggers can activate the stored energy as physiological symptoms in your mouth. Even though you experience physical symptoms as an individual, their underlying influences are relational, and ultimately collective.

Unhealed trauma can also be transmitted as intergenerational trauma passed through families both via family emotional or behavioral patterns, through DNA and as remembered experiences that are inherited in cells and systems of your mouth. There seems to be no limit, or geographic boundary, on how many generations the effects of famine, war or traumatic migration can be passed down from distant ancestors to descendants. Your teeth may be carrying the embodied energy of perhaps hundreds of years of trauma passed through genes and culture in families and social institutions. When you understand and work with this perspective, it becomes possible to address these generational patterns and increase your physical resilience.

My last root canal was in a lower right premolar carrying the archetype Rival, which flared up in my mid 40s when frustration at living with a group of friends prompted my third move in less than two years. As with several of my root canals, hindsight suggests that there was no physiological reason for the procedure. The sudden toothache wasn't caused by a cavity or abscess and didn't justify removing the nerve, but at the time I was unaware any alternative was possible.

I wish I could have read a book like this before my bad dental experiences had accumulated into such a high level of anxiety and mistrust that I started having panic attacks in the waiting room, in the dental chair and finally under general anaesthetic.

Woken from the anaesthetic with an incomplete root canal, I was sent home in confused tears and (kindly) told to sort myself out before coming back to finish off the procedure. I sought help from a hypnotherapist who stopped the panic attacks and incidentally loosened a straitjacket of powerlessness engendered by decades of dental trauma. A few weeks later I was able to return to the dental chair without freaking out.

No longer frozen in fear, I responded to my next bout of root pain a year or two later by looking for an alternative approach that could, and did, prevent another root canal. That's how I learned for the first time that teeth are dynamic, responsive and alive. They are connected to the body's ecosystem and capable of healing from the inside out.

I was amazed, delighted and very relieved to discover I could reverse tooth decay, relieve toothache and cure infection inside my own mouth with simple self-help remedies. For the next five years I immersed myself in 'alt oral' (alternative oral health) research and experimentation. I found out for the first time that dental check-ups could be pleasantly affirming instead of inevitably involving drilling, filling and billing.

Then, just before my 50th birthday I journaled a timeline of my unconventional life path, trying to make sense of the past so I could figure out what to do with my future. When I had the impulse to add my major dental crises to the timeline it was a revelation to see how each of my root canals coincided with, or followed, a stressful geographic uprooting. Soon after, I started natural oral health coaching as the Holistic Tooth Fairy.

My lifelong journey towards writing this book about the emotional influences on oral health has been pitted with root canals associated with periods of feeling rootless. This is not to say that anyone else's root canals are related to experiences of migration, moving house or travel! Each individual's mouth carries their own unique healing story, which weaves together life experiences, emotional patterns and family histories with wider cultural, environmental and historical influences.

I inherited flight as my default coping strategy and it took me until middle age to effectively start unpacking the complicated emotional baggage I carry about travel and migration. The inner work of self-awareness and spiritual practice I needed to do in order to settle down at last has been key to stabilizing my chronic oral health issues. Thus my work with the metaphysics of oral health which informs this book is inseparable from my family's roots and my life experiences.

Weaving roots

Three months before I was born, at the same time as the first adult molars were being seeded deep in my embryonic gums, my father persuaded my mother to emigrate from St Louis, USA to

Winnipeg, Canada, so he could avoid being drafted to fight the Vietnam War. That's how I came to be born on the unceded lands of the Anishinaabeg, Cree, Dakota, Dene, Metis and Oji-Cree Nations, far away from our extended family.

My parents named me Meliors, which comes from the same root as ameliorate, and means (among other things) making the world better through human endeavor. Throughout my life I have tried to help co-create a world in which oppressive structures and systems have no place or power, by using my intuition, my attention, my words and my hands to hold space for people to reconnect with the inner wisdom of their body.

Three years after I was born my father persuaded my mother to migrate again, this time literally to the other side of the world, for a job at Waikato University on the confiscated lands of the Tainui Confederation in Kirikiriroa, Hamilton in Aotearoa, New Zealand.

My father grew up Jewish, my mother grew up Baptist. But by the time they met each other they were both atheist, which is how I was raised, far away from any religious grand-parental influence. Nonetheless, comparative religion was a constant conversation throughout my childhood and I grew up with a strong spiritual curiosity. As soon as I understood the difference between atheist and agnostic, I identified myself as the latter in the first of many attempts to bridge the chasm between a skeptical, secular family culture and my personally undeniable awareness of the ineffable.

As a young adult I explored several spiritual traditions including contemporary versions of pan-European Wicca (which is when I first learned about healing with herbs) and various Western interpretations of Buddhism and Ayurveda, before eventually returning to my paternal roots with Reform and mystical flavors of Judaism.

Our family's international travels meant I attended eight different schools in four different countries. I left home at 16, then my hometown at 17 (just before my first root canal) and then became a single mother at 19. When my daughter was five we moved to the United States to connect with my extended family. While I was there a large cyst in my parotid salivary gland was surgically removed, leaving me with damaged nerves in my jaw and neck.

After two and a half years in the USA I returned to New Zealand for university (and a couple of unneeded and badly done root canals). After graduation I moved again to pursue a career in public policy which saw those recent root canals fail, get redone and ultimately be extracted, followed by a fourth root canal.

Not cut out for full-time office work, I burned out and broke down. Around that time my daughter left home and I suddenly found myself free of parental responsibility for the first time since my teens. I began to rebuild myself through energy healing, art and writing while travelling around New Zealand and Australia for five years. This adventure was unpleasantly punctuated with my fifth root canal.

Eventually I returned once more to my hometown of Hamilton, where I had my sixth and final root canal. That two-part surgery, which began with a panic attack under general anaesthetic, was a turning point. Within 18 months I was able to prevent what would have been my seventh root canal by researching and practicing what I now call an alt oral approach to understanding teeth and gums.

2.

A CABINET OF CURIOSITIES

Your mouth is a versatile vestibule: an intimate, private space but one where a stranger can easily glimpse the inside of your body. In the course of a few seconds it can turn from dark, humid and closed, to fully occupied with tasting, crushing and moving food, to open and airy with laughter.

As with other extra-sensitive body parts, you may simultaneously be preoccupied with your mouth's gross urges while remaining ignorant of its complex functions. Yet the more you know about the physical anatomy, physiology and biology of your mouth, the more effectively you can address your symptoms with energetic healing strategies. Abstract metaphysical interpretations are more meaningful when grounded in somatic awareness and close observation.

The body often tries to communicate emotional messages with subtle sensations that can escalate to agony if ignored. Most people have internalized the cultural disconnection between mouth and mind so thoroughly that they rarely notice anything untoward happening in their mouth except pain. But by the time your teeth or gums hurt, it can be difficult to identify, let alone respond effectively to the root cause

This chapter explains oral anatomy concepts, with imagery and language that will help you to understand how your body can heal teeth and gums. Dental interventions, as well as home remedies, are enhanced when you can picture, describe or affirm the physiological processes operating beyond your conscious awareness.

Teeth are dynamic, vibrant, living organisms and gums are multi-layered, complex combinations of bone, ligament and mucus membrane. Both respond quickly to all kinds of influences including what you eat, how you feel, what you think, or how stressed you are. This chapter gives you the vocabulary and concepts to fine-tune your conscious intentions for teeth and gum healing.

YOUR MULTI-TALENTED MOUTH

Your mouth is a master of multitasking (and not just when you talk with your mouth full). Whether you know it or not, your mouth is constantly juggling diverse roles in relation to your physical and metaphysical health.

Some of the mouth's jobs, like speaking, eating and drinking, usually happen in partnership with your conscious intentions. Other actions take place without any (or minimal) effort from your conscious mind but can be observed by you or other people, such as facial expressions or mouth breathing.

There is also a suite of additional activities that take place in time frames and spatial scales below the level of your awareness, such as the glacial movement of teeth and jawbones shaping your face or the diurnal cycles of your oral microbiome.

Your mouth is a communications switchboard, broadcasting speech, song and an array of expressive non-verbal sounds, mostly consciously controlled. Sometimes your mouth articulates thoughts that you didn't know you had. As I type these sentences I'm periodically aware of subvocalizing each word as I type it so that, without intending to, I'm whispering this book into existence.

Yet the communication goes two ways, inward as well as outwards. Your mouth sends pulses of pleasure or pain to your brain. When you take the first bite of a meal, your mouth sends signals (via the vagus nerve) to your stomach to start preparing for chewed food sliding down the hatch shortly.

Your mouth is a gateway, the biggest opening between the inside and outside of your body. It's the entrance to your digestive system, welcoming nourishment and hydration. Your mouth also provides access for less welcome visitors including externally sourced bacteria, fungi and viruses. These uninvited guests routinely hitch a ride on your food, drink or breath, not to mention anything, or anyone, you kiss, lick, suck or bite.

Your mouth can also be a threshold to deeply transformative inner work and emotional healing. Symptoms in your teeth and gums are the result of an interplay of physical and non-physical influences. This book's focus is on the latter, but before you flick ahead to the metaphysical interpretations, I invite you to spend a few minutes discovering more about the minerals, microbes and mechanics of your marvelous mouth.

Try this:
Gently twist the tip of your tongue
towards the back of your mouth.
Trace it over the arch of your upper palate.
Tuck it between your lower lip and front teeth.
Can you notice the different flavors
in each part of your mouth?
Perhaps the memory of a recent meal or toothpaste.
But also the utterly familiar taste of you.
Your own, unique, oral microbiome.

An oral inheritance

Long before your teeth became visible they were nestled inside your jaw, carrying a legacy that stretched back through generations. The DNA for your teeth was coded in the ovaries of your mother while she was inside your grandmother's body. Your first set of 24 baby teeth was initiated while you were in your mother's womb between six and eight weeks after conception, right about the time you were turning from an embryo into a fetus.

The permanent teeth (incisors, canines and premolars) that would eventually replace your baby teeth began their development between week 20 in utero and ten months after your birth. Your additional adult teeth were initiated between week 20 in utero (first molars) and five years of age (wisdom teeth).

If your mother was traumatized before your conception, or your grandmother was traumatized before your mother's conception, then your DNA may carry some impact of their trauma, expressed as stress hormones which disrupt immune, vascular, metabolic and endocrine systems, and can affect teeth development and oral health.

All this means that your teeth are influenced by your mother's pregnancy, your maternal grandmother's pregnancy, and their lives prior to those pregnancies, which in turn were influenced by their own mothers and grandmothers going back generation after generation.

But it's not only the maternal lineage that influences your oral health. Teeth may also carry the impact of trauma from your father's and grandfathers' lives, sometimes going back many generations as well. A father with unhealed trauma may produce sperm with altered DNA expression which can affect their offspring's developing cells, including teeth (Costa et al).

The oral microbiome you have now was seeded during birth, with bacteria picked up from your passage through the birth canal. (Babies born by caesarean section miss out on this bacterial inheritance which also populates skin, gut and genital microbiomes). Your oral microbiome was further populated by everything that you sucked, gummed or licked, mostly in the first few hours, to a lesser extent over the following days, and occasionally during the following years.

Very few of the types of bacteria living in your adult oral microbiome arrived later than early childhood. Most of your oral bacteria now are still the same as your mother's or other early caregiver's. Your oral microbiome's resilience or vulnerability to gum disease or tooth decay is heavily influenced by your ancestors and your parents, your birth experience and your infancy.

THE TEETH–BRAIN CONNECTION

Baby teeth (aka milk or deciduous teeth) start to appear when most of us are a few months old and start falling out in the same order from age five. Adult teeth usually grow into the spaces left by baby teeth, starting at the front and gradually extending to the back of your mouth with the teeth that should last the rest of your life.

At birth your newborn brain is still incomplete and as different parts of the brain (cortex) develop they have a mutually influential relationship with the teeth that develop at the same time. Dr Christian Beyer associates the eruption of each tooth with a psychological stage of development in brain function and structure.

Nearly ninety percent of your brain development took place between birth and your third birthday and, just like your teeth, your brain was influenced by both genetics (inherited potential) and the influence of your environment (especially interactions with your primary caregiver). As a newborn, you were utterly dependent on your mother, father or other caregivers as the biological regulators of your immature physiological and emotional systems (Maté).

Your physiological system established neural pathways and hormonal responses before you learned to talk. Up to a million new synapses (nerve connections) were being established every second in response to emotional interactions that stimulated the release of hormones. Happy, safe, loving experiences released endorphins, which encouraged the growth and connection of synapses.

Stressful, scary or frustrating experiences that were not quickly resolved with loving connection instead activated stress hormones such as cortisol, which inhibited the growth, or even caused shrinkage, of parts of your brain. What is usually referred to as personality can in fact be understood mostly as patterns of adaption to your earliest experiences (Maté).

The patterns of adaption imprinted on your developing cortex can also be imprinted into your developing teeth.

Extracting the abusers

Lizzie[1] was six when she tripped on a flagstone floor and smashed her top front teeth. Her parents had divorced a couple of years earlier because her mother had had an affair with the man who became Lizzie's stepfather. Lizzie hoped the accident would make her ugly enough that her stepfather would stop sexually abusing her, and her mother would stop acting jealous.

Tooth 8, the Nurturer archetype, died first. Lizzie's mother maintained a polished public persona of white privilege but behind closed doors she inflicted physical, sexual and psychological abuse. Lizzie took the brunt of her mother's mistreatment to try to protect her younger siblings.

Tooth 9, the Leader archetype, died a few years later around the time that her father remarried and Lizzie lost all hope that his benign neglect could provide respite from her mother's abuse.

Lizzie hid her rebellious spirit because her mother obliterated

---

1   All names have been changed to protect confidentiality and all client stories are shared with permission.

her sense of self and her stepmother forbade it. Lizzie had to be silent, wanted to be invisible, tried to stay small and hoped to go unnoticed. She felt nothing but resigned to enduring a fathomless pit of never-ending sorrow. When she was eleven both top front teeth were given root canals and eventually she carried a mouthful of crowns and fillings, needing treatment for cracks, infections and an abscess.

Then in her thirties Lizzie started what would be years of therapy and personal growth, and blossomed into a cycle-breaking mother, healer and writer. I met her nearly 70 years after the original trauma, when she needed to have the infected front teeth pulled to make way for implants after achieving remission from cancer.

"I'm tired of surprises," she said. "I want my body to finally be happy."

She found good dental professionals in neighboring towns, but at first lying back in the dental chair felt just like being a child waiting for the next episode of abuse.

As I coached Lizzie through a lengthy dental treatment plan, she chose not to endure the tension and fear by shutting down, as she had learned to do as a child. Instead, she used many of the insights and exercises described in this book to enable her mouth to become a conduit for healing the childhood abuse.

At the end of a long year of successful dental surgeries she told me that having her front teeth extracted had been like removing the abusers from her mouth. Receiving the implants felt like a door opening to a new life.

Living layers

Try this:
Slowly run your tongue
along the inside arch of your upper jaw.
Can you feel the bulbous curved surfaces
of each back tooth?

The elegant concave of each front tooth?
Lightly tap your lower teeth against your upper teeth.
Can you feel the percussive clack
resonating in your ears?

I spent most of my life under the impression that my teeth were lumps of stone, as lifeless as nails or hair. In fact, teeth are complex, multi-layered ecosystems, alive with pulsing nerves in the pulp, fluids flowing through the dentin and constantly renewing enamel.

Healthy enamel is the hardest, most mineralized, substance in the body: calcium hydroxyapatite crystals make up 87% of the enamel (along with phosphorus, magnesium and potassium). Enamel bears the brunt of biting and chewing.

Underneath the enamel is a softer layer of dentin, a more bone-like substance that extends down inside the alveolar part of the jawbone or socket. Both enamel and dentin are made from crystal fibers packed into tubules (rods) projecting between the tooth surface and the central pulp. These tubules pump remineralizing fluids outwards from the pulp to the enamel.

The pulp chamber tapers from the center of each tooth to the tip of every root, full of tissues, blood and nerves. Pulp is the tender heart and mind of each tooth, protected by the crystalline mineral layers surrounding it. Pulp can send information back to your brain via nerves in the form of sensations (cold! pain!). But mostly it conveys the body's nutrients, fluids, oxygen, proteins and hormones into your teeth to reinforce and repair the hardworking outer layers.

Dentinal flow

Try this:
Place your first two fingers just under your ears.
Massage lightly behind the corners of your lower jaw.
Does the massage stimulate
a gush of saliva into your mouth?

You are activating your parotid glands, which hang down the sides of your neck like big dangling earrings. The parotid glands produce saliva and the hormones that drive dentinal flow. Dentinal flow is the mechanism that powers tooth and jawbone remineralization and gum regeneration. It is the main engine maintaining strong, resilient, shiny, white teeth and tight pink gums.

In healthy circumstances, remineralization naturally happens all the time.

Plants draw up raw minerals from the earth through their roots and convert them into bio-available nutrients, which you may consume directly as vegetables or further along the food chain as animal products. Once in your digestive system, the minerals in your food get separated out from the fibers, fluids and other nutrients. Calcium, phosphorus, magnesium, potassium as well as traces of silica, iron and other minerals are carried in your blood up to your jaw.

Dentinal flow pumps a mineral-rich fluid into the tooth roots and then outwards from the pulp, through the dentin, to repair and maintain the enamel. As fluids travel through the layers inside your teeth, needed nutrients get deposited in the pulp and the dentin until all that is left is a pure mineral solution of calcium hydroxyapatite and phosphorus combined into calcium phosphate.

Drop by microscopic drop, your enamel is regenerated and restored with calcium phosphate, like a stalagmite grows from drops of limestone-saturated water. The constantly renewing mineral surface of healthy teeth helps to repel bacterial films such as plaque and its calcification into tartar.

However, dentinal-flow-driven remineralization can be switched off whenever your stress (or blood sugar) levels get too high. When cortisone and other stress hormones flood your body, they switch off non-essential organs and glands, including the parotid. They constrict muscles, the flow of blood and other fluids. Cortisone also causes vascular changes in tooth pulp, which inhibit the flow of fluids. When stress switches off your dentinal flow, the nutrients in even the healthiest diet can't get to where they are needed to maintain your teeth and gums (Akcali et al).

Gum tissues

The gum includes four main types of periodontal tissue: alveolar bone, periodontal ligament, cementum, and gingiva. Each type of tissue plays a physiological role in the overall mouth system. These physiological roles can be seen as parallel to psychological roles. Symptoms in these tissues are the embodiment of emotional, spiritual or psychological adaptations to stressors, as described in Chapter 10.

Alveolar bone is the thin ridge of jawbone that surrounds each tooth with a bony socket. The role of the alveolar bone is to be a foundation that nurtures new teeth and supports tooth roots to grow and stand firm and straight.

Periodontal ligaments are strong stretchy fibers that surround each tooth root like a sling. The role of the periodontal ligaments is to be flexible shock absorbers, so that you can move your mouth freely without destabilizing your teeth through eating, speaking and expressing.

Cementum is made up of microscopic sticky threads that connect teeth roots to the mass of periodontal ligaments, tightly binding the border between gum and tooth.

Gingiva is the visible surface of your gums, a wet pink permeable membrane which covers all the rest of the periodontal tissue. The role of the gingiva is to protect and contain the nerves, blood vessels, lymph, facia, muscles and bone of the jaws and be a biological habitat for oral bacteria to carry out their diverse roles.

SENSITIVE NERVES

Have you ever wondered why toothache hurts so badly or why teeth can feel so uncomfortably sensitive to temperature? The heightened sensations in your mouth are the result of more nerve endings concentrated into that relatively small area than (almost) any other part of your body.

Tiny, threadlike nerves ending in the pulp at the center of each tooth send signals through a dense tangle of thicker nerves that travel along the jaw to carry sensory information just a few centimeters to the receptors in your back brain.

There in your motor cortex, fully one third of the brain's sensory receptors are connected to the nerves in and around your mouth and jaw. Some of the influx of information received via these nerves is translated into *conscious* perceptions of movement or pressure, taste, texture or temperature, pleasure or pain.

However, the most crucial information sent from the nerves in your mouth is largely *unconscious* and indicates safety or threat. Your conscious mind is rarely aware of grinding your teeth after a tense day, of biting or sucking in your lips when you aren't comfortable speaking up, or of jutting your chin out to appear braver than you feel. These subtle patterns of movement (which you probably started doing before you could talk) are picked up by your nerves, which tell your brain that you don't feel safe.

When you feel under threat, your body produces stress hormones including adrenaline and cortisol, which activate a range of survival mechanisms affecting the mouth (as well as the rest of the body). Blood and dentinal flow are diverted from your teeth and gums to your jaw muscles. Energy supplies are mobilized in the form of sugar molecules into your blood and saliva, increasing the acidity of your oral microbiome.

The stress hormone cortisol mobilizes calcium from bones and teeth to circulate it back into the blood stream. This means that an excess of cortisol can demineralize and weaken teeth and jaw bones. It can reduce the height of alveolar bone, which contributes to receding gums and can undermine the stability of teeth.

So although you may be brushing and flossing like a boss, if you are in the habit of unconsciously moving your mouth in ways that signal 'I'm not feeling safe', then the physiological systems that maintain your teeth and gums aren't able to work properly.

Suck it up

Two main saliva ducts sit under your tongue, which is why saliva tends to accumulate just behind your front bottom teeth (not by coincidence one of the most common areas for plaque to calcify). Two more major ducts are located inside your cheeks. And because nature likes redundancies, there are several more minor ducts dotted around your mouth.

A dry mouth is the body's response to fear and can also occur as a side effect from stress-relieving medications. Dry mouth inhibits the natural production of saliva, which is your mouth's primary defense against bacteria. Thus, any reduction in saliva may mean an increased risk of tooth decay, periodontal disease and oral infections.

Try this:
Gently push your tongue to one side, between the
nubbly chewing surface of your molars,
to explore the inside of your cheek.
Can you feel a tiny, soft bump like a painless pimple
in the middle of that stretchy wet wall?
That is a saliva duct and stroking it with the tip of
your tongue may be enough to stimulate a gush of spit.
If not, try sucking your cheeks against the outside of
your teeth while thinking about biting into a lemon.

3.

A MANIFESTO
FOR METAPHYSICAL HEALING

I've evolved the following principles over years of coaching hundreds of clients. This manifesto is a signpost at the intersection where physical symptoms and remedies, and dental diagnoses and interventions, encounter emotional, psychological, or ancestral influences and respond to energetic, somatic or spiritual insights.

The following principles are intended to act as guard rails to help keep you safe as you apply metaphysical theories to individual experiences.

1. Feel what your body is telling you

The single most important skill for anyone to cultivate in a metaphysical approach to oral health is somatic awareness: observing internal sensations in your own body, including very subtle feelings. By the time your body has escalated to spontaneous sensations of extreme discomfort or pain, your symptoms may be too advanced for metaphysical healing to work without the need for dental interventions.

You may be used to inspecting your mouth for discoloration, holes in enamel or swollen gums but sight is a limited sense when self-evaluating internal issues.

As you read through this book, and especially if you try the exercises, you may feel a physical reaction in your mouth or the rest of your body. Pay attention to what you're reading if your body responds with pangs of sensitivity shooting through your teeth, tingling extremities or whole body shaking, laughter, yawning, tears, or an impulse to move. These are normal responses, so let them move through you, observe with relaxed curiosity and take note.

Try this:
Close your lips and breathe gently through your nose
as you answer the following questions.
What do you feel inside your mouth right now?
What is the tip of your tongue touching?
Are your upper and lower teeth touching,
at the front and back, on the left and right?
What is the taste of your mouth right now?
Is there any sensation of movement
such as a tingle or a throb?
What is the temperature in your mouth?
Is there a particular part of your mouth
with more sensation than the rest?

You may be used to interpreting what you observe in your mouth using logic, but this time, ask yourself what emotions are present as you pay attention to physical sensations.

Focus on the physical sensation of your emotion,
where does it feel strongest?
Visualize the emotion,

imaging its color, size and texture.
Is it moving around?
Is its movement fast or slow, smooth or jerky?
Does the emotion remind you of a being or a place?
Does it have an age?
Does it feel connected to someone in your family?
Does it change as you pay attention to it?

Somatic awareness takes curiosity, stillness and practice. Over the coming days, try to pay attention to how you feel when you use your mouth to eat, speak, sing or breathe. What do you feel when you brush or floss your teeth? When do you feel a shock of sensitivity? Are you aware of subtle sensations that aren't quite sensitivity? If you feel discomfort, observe it closely to determine whether it's a dull ache or a sharp pain.

Ground your observations by making notes, as words or images. Start a fresh page or a fresh notebook, scrawl notes in the margin of this book or type them into your phone. Keep track of your observations because subjective sensations are often fleeting and ambiguous. Making notes and looking back at them later will help you start to make sense of your metaphysical themes, patterns or cycles.

Build your capacity to understand and trust what your body is telling you by responding to its needs. When you feel hungry, eat what makes your body feel good. When you feel tired, pause and rest. When you have an urge to move your body, stand, stretch, walk, dance or play.

Try asking your mouth a question (like 'what do you need?') and pay attention to any physical sensations as you say the question and think about possible answers. This can be an especially valuable exercise when you are struggling to make a decision about a dental intervention.

2. Respond pragmatically

One of the most powerful effects of working with metaphysical meanings of teeth and gums is to improve your experience of any necessary dental procedures and their outcomes. Understanding and responding to the underlying energetic influences on your symptoms can help you to prevent complications such as ongoing infections, failed fillings or root canals, cavitations, implant rejections and all the other things that can go wrong with dental surgeries.

In many cases it may be possible to repair and restore your teeth and gums with a holistic approach that includes metaphysical strategies. However, more often than not, by the time you prioritize this kind of healing, it's too late to avoid a dental procedure altogether. Metaphysical strategies are most useful when used to complement physical strategies of holistic home care and conservative dental support.

Despite anecdotes of spontaneous regrowth of teeth and gums, for most people in most circumstances, relying solely on metaphysical healing for advanced symptoms is not realistic. Don't be disheartened though.

There are still benefits from understanding and responding to what your symptoms are trying to tell you. There are bullets to be dodged. You could get a smaller filling than you might have needed otherwise. You could get a big filling instead of a root canal. You could cure mild gingivitis without it escalating to periodontal disease. You could stabilize receding gums and avoid bone loss enough to stop teeth falling out.

It is probably more realistic to aim to make your next dental intervention the last one. When necessary, act fast to stabilize your body with the surgical repair it needs and then continue to work on preventing any further deterioration.

3. THE MAP IS NOT THE TERRITORY

Part II describes six systems of metaphysical associations including tooth-by-tooth meanings as well as more generalized symptom correlations. All these methods should be understood as starting points for interpretation. They provide questions, rather than answers. They offer a vocabulary that can help you begin to make sense of the 'why' behind your oral health issues.

But, if you have ever landed somewhere where you don't speak the language, you know the limits of knowing only a few words when trying to have a nuanced conversation. With the right vocabulary you might be able to buy a ticket or find the bathroom but to talk about anything substantial you also need good grammar, intelligible pronunciation and the kind of speed that comes with familiarity.

Helpful as they can be, these metaphysical frameworks will only take you so far in understanding the underlying influences on your teeth. When it comes to the emotional landscape of your mouth, metaphysical associations are most useful as signposts. To have an in-depth, meaningful and ultimately healing understanding of your teeth and gums symptoms, you need to develop a conversational practice with your body.

4. EXPLORE WITH RELAXED CURIOSITY

Relaxed curiosity is a type of calm, kind attention in which you are open to whatever comes into your awareness. It is unattached to any particular outcome, or the need to make sense of what happens. It can be hard to access the quality of relaxed curiosity when you are suffering pain or anxiety, but it's worth remembering to try anyway.

Relaxed curiosity is the opposite of trying to confirm your assumptions or seeking a universally applicable explanation. Those kinds of rigid thinking, whether entrenched in scientific skepticism or naïve new age credulity, can prevent you from understanding and engaging with your unique combination of needs and circumstances.

Avoid applying a literal interpretation of any metaphysical framework to your own situation. Be especially careful about how you interpret anyone else's symptoms or experiences (or how you allow anyone else to interpret your symptoms).

Try this:
Imagine meeting your mouth
as though finding a dear friend in distress,
who is unable or unwilling to tell you why.
First make sure they are safe right now,
that their urgent physical needs for water, food,
warmth and rest are being met:
do this for your own physical needs.
Then imagine sitting patiently
with your mouth-friend,
offering them unconditional support,
making it clear that you are willing to listen
when they are ready to speak
but just as willing to never know what's going on.
Imagine drawing on every instinct
and bit of shared history
to help them feel safe and trusting.
Hang out with them, let them lead the conversation,
don't give up and don't make demands.

5. Tell your own story (and hold it lightly)

Your life history has left an energetic imprint on your teeth and gums of emotional associations, psychological patterns and ancestral influences, which should be understood as stories rather than literal facts.

The interpretive frameworks described in this book are best used as prompts to develop stories drawn from your own experience and history. Focus on the associations that resonate most for you and leave aside the rest. The real power of metaphysical healing comes through culturally relevant metaphors, personally meaningful images and themes that expand your self-understanding.

As a human, you are simultaneously much like all other humans in some ways and unique in other ways. You are the best person to make sense of the emotional landscape of your mouth because no one else has the same combination of emotional patterns, old traumas, environmental influences, family histories or dental experiences embodied into their teeth and gums as you do.

Storytelling and your imagination are powerful tools for healing. The brain can release the same hormones or trigger the same physiological functions in response to an imaginary situation as it does in response to reality.

Some of the ways you can use the metaphysical frameworks in Part II to develop and work with your own healing story include:

- Focus for meditation.
- Talking points for therapy, coaching or deep conversation.
- Prompts for journal writing (see the appendix).
- Dream work in your sleep.
- Inspiration for art that expresses and explores these themes.
- Intellectual integration with other frameworks such as personality types or astrology.

Finding your healing story through these practices can give you a delicate, imaginative tool for healing in private, in which it doesn't matter whether you are drawing on your own memories, your imagination, transgenerational memories, popular culture or past life visions. It is likely that your healing story will change and evolve over time, as you release layers of old hurts and move through transformative insights.

Healing stories are not historical facts, which doesn't detract from their usefulness in transforming your personal relationship with your oral health. Unless you are planning to share your story in public, there's no need to get bogged down with the accuracy of the images, scenes or feelings that inform your healing story.

But be careful! It can be intoxicating to finally make sense of your symptoms with a compelling metaphysical interpretation. That excitement can lead you to give your healing story more weight than a fragile web of imagination, ancestral or past life interpretations can hold.

Never rush to use your healing story to define your public identity and be extra cautious about mentioning any stories involving other people. Consider carefully whether there is any therapeutic benefit in sharing your healing story, and if the potential benefit outweighs the risks.

At this point in history there are no external filters left between your impulse to share and the possibility of global reach. Before you take your healing story out of the safe space of your healing work (e.g. your journal or a confidential conversation) ensure you are very certain about what *is* actually true and be prepared to deal with other people's responses.

6. Accept no shame and assign no blame

Have you internalized the widespread public discourse that shames dental patients (or their parents) for symptoms? Do you believe dental problems occur solely because you don't floss enough, you drink too much soda, or you breastfeed at night? Such victim-blaming perspectives can easily taint the application of metaphysical frameworks to oral health.

However, there is a world of difference between taking the blame for your symptoms versus recognizing that you can be an active participant in transforming your healing story.

Metaphysical explanations most effectively support healing when you assume that you (and everyone else) were doing your best in circumstances constrained by fundamental conflicts between the needs of our physical and emotional selves. You have inherited your ancestors' physical patterns of adaption to historical conflicts, and also adapted physically to the particular challenges of your lifetime.

The time, place and people you were born into, and the particular circumstances of life that you have navigated, have been shaped by the forces of colonialism or imperialism and capitalism or communism. These vast social systems are experienced differently depending on where you are on the planet and on the axes of gender, race, class, sexuality, ability, age and generation and so on. This is all just as true for anyone else as it is for you, including your parents and your dentists.

There should be no shame in having learned survival patterns (such as jaw clenching) that impacted your oral health. There should be no shame for not having identified emotional patterns sooner, or for finding it difficult to interrupt those patterns consistently once you've recognized them. There should certainly be no shame in encountering an old healing story or emotional pattern when it shows up *again*, this time in your mouth.

Show yourself and others compassion and generosity as you make sense of your healing stories.

7. EMBRACE THE ABSURD AND LEAN INTO RESISTANCE

The process of metaphysical healing can sometimes feel like ricocheting between dramatic emotional highs and lows. It could stir up unwelcome insights that rock your foundations or unpleasant memories you thought you'd worked through already.

Yet your teeth and gums thrive on joy, play, pleasure and silliness. Many of the emotional patterns that your mouth embodies as symptoms were started when you were a very small child, and small children are easily amused.

As you map metaphysical interpretations onto your symptoms there may be puns, caricatures, ridiculous blind spots, over-the-top fears, outrageous assumptions and weirdly inexplicable jokes. Enjoy a light-hearted approach to healing and be willing to laugh at yourself. Laughter is a massage for your mouth.

You may also feel uncomfortable emotions such as anger, grief or shame, but first you could encounter resistance. Resistance can look like denial, avoidance, or procrastination. It can feel like numbness, blankness, an edgy urge to escape or to change the subject.

Your resistance has been an active partner in your health and survival for so long that it's implicated in your particular symptoms. The experience of resistance is there to protect you from something that subconsciously feels more risky than the symptoms in your teeth and gums. Allow yourself space to observe and explore your resistance, fear or need for control, rather than trying to push past to the 'real' work.

Sandy is a single mother and a music therapist, who is comfortable working with the metaphysical aspects of whole body health both for herself and her clients. She came to me with tooth and jaw pain, and obsessive dental anxiety. In our first session, she became aware of internal feelings of resistance to working on her oral health, which she addressed with self-directed reiki.

Resistance reappeared in our fifth coaching session after Sandy filled me in on the main events since we had last met. Her two brothers had come to town to stage an intervention with their alcoholic mother, with whom Sandy had a close but very difficult relationship. Despite her brothers' support, Sandy was left feeling ashamed that the situation remained unresolved. She felt unworthy and overwhelmed as the caretaking daughter.

Three days before our session, while working intently with one of her own therapy clients, Sandy clenched her teeth so hard that the back of her left jaw locked up for two days of intense discomfort and fear that seemed to undo all the improvements of our earlier work together.

I began to guide Sandy through a self-massage for her jaw, asking her to move slowly and attend to all the sensations, emotions and thoughts that came into her awareness as she gently touched her face. Sandy kept trying to rush ahead with the massage but I kept reminding her to slow down.

After a few minutes she remarked that the middle finger of her right hand had become so sore and stiff that she could hardly continue the massage. I switched focus to this finger, asking her to cradle it lovingly in her left hand, where she identified the energy of resistance in that finger, which now felt sprained.

Middle fingers are on the pericardium meridian, which extends behind the wisdom teeth (i.e. the part of her jaw where Sandy had been feeling pain all weekend). The meridian is named for the sac of tough, fibrous tissue that wraps around the heart to protect it from injury. In traditional Chinese medicine this meridian is associated with feeling unlovable, unworthy and ashamed, emotions which were triggered intensely for Sandy by the recent family intervention with her mother.

As Sandy focused on where she felt the resistance, the feelings changed under our relaxed curious attention. Sensations of discomfort started jumping around her body like a smart, scared, playful three-year-old so we played its game of hide-and-seek with patient compassion until the sensations dissipated.

Resistance had been one of Sandy's survival strategies since she was a toddler. It helped to protect her tender heart from a lack of maternal love and emotional connection in her childhood. Paying attention with relaxed curiosity helped the toddler pattern of resistance learn to trust that adult-Sandy would keep her safe while feeling shame, disappointment or anger.

After our session, Sandy started an art project to make portraits of the feelings of resistance and shame. When we met again a month later the toothache was gone, and she told me she was not obsessing about her teeth anymore.

8. Harness the power of placebo

A placebo is anything that seems like a medical treatment (such as a sugar pill) but doesn't contain an active substance meant to affect health. A person can have a perceived or actual physical response to a placebo, either symptoms improving or what appear to be side effects.

The main theory explaining the placebo effect is that it's the result of a person's belief in the treatment's benefit and their expectation of feeling better (Marchant). However, a placebo effect can occur even when the subject is skeptical or knows they are taking a 'dummy' remedy. Researchers speculate that placebo effects occur when the rituals of taking 'medication', exercise, eating well or other self-care activities are enhanced by quality emotional awareness and attention (Arnold).

A skeptical but willing approach to metaphysical healing can be a way to harness and direct the power of active and self-aware placebo effects. Metaphysical healing works best when you take responsibility for your own healing to proactively and persistently experiment to find the unique combination of nutrition, hygiene and exercise that works best for you. It rests on a foundation of consistent meditation, visualization, affirmation, and your own most effective energy healing modalities. This is definitely not the same thing as waiting and wishing for your symptoms to disappear so you can go back to your regular life!

You may be able to harness the placebo effect by courageously sitting with uncomfortable emotions, challenging cherished beliefs, changing ingrained habits (sometimes turning your life upside down in the process) and making empowered decisions about dental procedures.

9. Healing is a Practice, not an Outcome

The emotional patterns imprinted on your teeth and gums have been operating unconsciously for years, sometimes generations. It can take weeks, months or longer to release them and embed new patterns in their place.

Your intention may be to avoid fillings in your teeth, but that's not an end point. You can remineralize decay and get the all clear from the dentist this year, but next year that tooth, or another, may present you with decay showing another layer of energetic hurt that needs to be released. So healing, prevention and maintenance are a lifelong project.

You may think surely you've done enough work, and then your body will draw your attention to where you are not finished. It may never be fully resolved. You may be healing for the rest of your life. This is my personal experience and I've been doing this with my teeth for more than ten years.

However, as you come back again and again to attend to the underlying metaphysical needs of your body the symptoms can become milder, less frequent, and faster to release. The true miracle of metaphysical self-healing is not the complete cure, but the sense of empowered sovereignty over your body.

The qualities that enable your healing, that help to release the symptoms, relieve discomfort and bring your body into balance are qualities that improve your life. It's a win-win approach to reduce stress, enjoy more pleasure, be connected in community and above all to be mindful and present in your body. Living your life this way can not only improve your oral health, it can also improve your general health, your mental health, and your emotional well-being.

Part II:
An Atlas

The parents have eaten sour grapes and the children's teeth are set on edge.

Jer. 31:29; Ezek. 18:2

4.

MAPPING THE LANDSCAPE OF YOUR MOUTH

The mouth mapping frameworks in this part of the book layer holographic representations of your energetic, emotional and spiritual selves onto the physical landscape of your mouth.

Within the limited and obscure literature that explores the metaphysical meanings of oral health there are two complementary approaches to mapping the mouth: mouth meridians and tooth types. In both approaches metaphysical associations work with different parts of the mouth whether or not there are symptoms present.

I usually find the tooth type approaches most useful as their metaphysical interpretations are logically consistent with dental charts. Tooth type themes stay coherent at various scales, from quadrants of the mouth to individual tooth surfaces, allowing you to change your focus, like a dynamic digital map of a small town.

But the first, fundamental, and foundational approach to metaphysical mapping is the system of mouth meridians (better known as teeth meridians), which is based on traditional Chinese medicine concepts. The mouth meridian system applies emotional associations to specific locations in the mouth by linking them to a whole body system of energy channels.

The mouth meridian channels meander around the mouth like prehistoric paths, surfacing at specific locations like settlements that seem almost dreamlike in their distance from today's built environment. Like archaeologists interpreting landscape-sized calendars, working with mouth meridians can require you to traverse an imaginative bridge across a cultural divide.

Meridian origins

Although there are some questions about the historical authenticity of traditional Chinese medicine (TCM), there is archeological evidence that elements of what is now known as TCM have been practiced for millennia. Acupuncture needles have been found in Han Dynasty tombs (206 BCE–220 CE) and there are written descriptions of Chinese diagnostic techniques dated from around 400 BCE.

For most of its history TCM was only accessible to the affluent ruling classes of Chinese society, who favored it until about 1850 when Western medicine began to overtake TCM there, after some Chinese doctors returned from studying medicine outside of the country. A hundred years later, TCM was consolidated and systemized as part of Mao Zedong's efforts to unite China behind traditional Chinese values. Today TCM is available alongside, but not usually recognized as valid by, Western medicine throughout China (Chu).

Acupuncture is the element of TCM with the longest history outside of China, dating back to the mid-seventeenth century. Since the People's Republic of China began opening up to the West in 1972, other elements of TCM including Chinese herbal medicine, tongue and iris diagnoses and reflexology have become popular internationally as well.

There seems to be little evidence that the meridian system of TCM as practiced in China extended to teeth until the 1960s. From that point Western researchers using electroacupuncture began to identify and decode mutual correlations between the meridian energy channels used in acupuncture and their respective adjacent teeth (Gleditsch).

How meridians interact with teeth

In TCM, strong emotions are believed to disrupt the normal flow of qi (energy) along the meridian channels. Anger pushes qi upwards, fear drives qi downwards and worry causes stagnation. Teeth are just one of the many places in the body where meridians are affected by physiological expressions of emotions.

Unconsciously repeated micro-movements affect your mouth meridians in a similar way that a habitual frown or smile eventually imprints wrinkles into the skin of your face. Your most frequent facial expressions and tones of voice are physiological expressions of the emotional patterns that form your personality.

As you experience and express emotional states with varying degrees of consciousness, they affect the way your teeth and tongue interact with the sensitive meridian points. Your unique speech patterns imprint on the meridians via the repeated vibrations from your voice box and position of your tongue, lips and cheeks as they form the vowel and consonant sounds of your vocalizations.

Thus, a muttered self-deprecation when you've made a mistake, a daily routine of nagging your children, or the 'yes' you say when you want to say 'no', each create a specific profile or pattern of pressure onto the meridian points.

Introducing new habits of speaking truthfully, smiling with compassion, or expressing your authentic self wholeheartedly can alter the patterns of pressure on your meridians, change the energy flow in your mouth and support your oral health.

Meridians are also stimulated on a level below conscious

perception by the pulsing of nerves in the tooth pulp, the subtle electrical charge of calcium hydroxyapatite crystals on the surface of the enamel, and the flow of dentinal fluids through the dentin. Dentinal flow runs in circadian rhythms, so meridians are easily able to adapt to their temporary absence or restriction due to stress. However, chronic stress inhibits dentinal flow over an extended period (see Chapter 2) potentially causing long-term effects on the adjacent meridians.

Dental interventions and meridians

When a tooth has been filled, crowned or capped it is still able to touch nearby meridians, so they continue to be massaged by conscious and subconscious movements and vocalizations. Underneath a filling, dentinal flow continues to pump nutrients into the rest of the tooth and its central nerves still pulse with hormonal information. However, the dentinal flow and crystalline electric charge of the tooth enamel may be more or less compromised depending on the size of the filling, crown or cap.

Orthodontic braces, mouthguards and other dental appliances, as well as jewelry inside the mouth such as grills or piercings, can all change the way that mouth meridians are stimulated by movement and sound. They may also form a barrier between a healthy tooth and its adjacent meridian.

A stable root-canaled tooth, a biocompatible implant or a well-fitted denture will allow the larger muscle movements and vocal vibrations of your mouth to activate your meridians. However, without nerves, dentinal tubules and all, or most, of the crystalline tooth enamel, the nearest meridians won't receive the same subtle stimuli that intact teeth provide.

The gap left by an extraction that isn't replaced by an implant or denture means there is no direct stimulation for the pulled tooth's adjacent meridians, due to the lack of gross movements and subtle energies.

However, your energy body is incredibly resilient. The meridian system has multiple redundancies so that if one point of stimulation in the mouth is compromised, the rest of the system can adapt. Each meridian is present in every quadrant of the mouth and in touch with at least four individual teeth. The meridians also cross the upper and lower palate and are massaged by your tongue as you breathe, eat, drink or speak.

Meridian channels extend throughout the rest of the body, from your toes to your fingertips, and they are stimulated by the movements of your hands and feet as much as they are by your mouth and jaw. There are many places on the body where meridians rise to the surface and can be deliberately therapeutically activated. Acupuncture, acupressure, reflexology and emotional freedom techniques (EFT) are just some of the modalities that engage with the meridian system.

Thus, most individual dental interventions usually have a very limited impact on the meridian system as a whole (unless there is an infection or other complication). Even multiple procedures or extensive tooth loss can be compensated by consciously maintaining the meridian system in the rest of your body.

Getting Oriented in Your Mouth

Because the meridians are located in the soft tissue of the mouth and not the teeth themselves, I have started calling them mouth meridians, rather than the widely used term teeth meridians. However, to apply the meridian's emotional associations in your own metaphysical healing it helps to identify where each tooth is sitting in your jaw so you can identify which pair of meridians is closest to your symptoms.

A tooth that is in a non-standard position (due to orthodontic treatment, tooth loss or some other reason) may be closest to a different meridian pair than shown on most teeth meridian charts.

Meridians use a different mapping method than the tooth type and tooth archetype systems in which psychosocial associations are intrinsic to each kind of tooth, no matter where it is sitting in your mouth. If you have teeth that have shifted around in your mouth, you'll need to apply both these frameworks with discretion.

To start mapping metaphysical interpretations onto your symptoms you'll need to know which individual tooth, type of tooth or gum location to reference. If you aren't sure, ask your dentist to share a copy of your dental chart (see the note about dental chart numbering in the Introduction).

Tooth type origins

What I call tooth type approaches were developed around the turn of this century by European dentists who have combined their clinical experience with esoteric studies (unfortunately their work is not yet available in English translation). Dr Michèle Caffin and Dr Christian Beyer have each developed their own comprehensive and detailed systems of metaphysical meanings for teeth based on clinical observations. Their distinctive approaches offer psychological and interpersonal interpretations that are specific to each type of tooth, each individual tooth and (with Beyer) even specific surfaces of each tooth.

Dr Christian Beyer, a clinical dentist and homeopath, observed patterns of decay in his patients that could not be explained by bacteria alone. He noticed identical cavities develop in teeth that were not adjacent but rather, were on the same type of tooth located in different quadrants. This led him to develop a framework of 'dental decoding' (now renamed psychoneurodontology), which connects the universal chronological order of teeth emergence with brain development.

Each tooth has a metaphysical association that Dr Beyer argues is influenced by the part of the brain that was developing at the same time as the tooth because each tooth's nerve endings (inside the pulp) are connected to particular sensory motor receptors in the brain.

Dr Michèle Caffin, a dentist and acupuncturist, has written extensively about the psychological, emotional and spiritual influences on oral health she has observed in 35 years of clinical practice. She also associates each tooth with different mystical tools including astrology and the Kabbalah.

I am indebted to Dr Beyer's and Dr Caffin's books for inspiring and informing the development of my own metaphysical framework of Tooth Archetypes. As I laboriously translated their theories for my own education I also experimented with adapting them to practical application. In doing so I incorporated intersectional awareness and trauma-informed interpretations to meet the needs of my diverse clients.

However, it was through my client work (even before reading Beyer) that I began associating each tooth with an archetype. I gradually developed my own vocabulary for naming and describing metaphysical associations for all the elements of the mouth from its quadrants to the teeth, to layers of gum tissue and more. In doing so I have both consolidated and expanded existing tooth type and mouth meridians approaches, into the frameworks described in the following chapters, which I hope my readers find consistent, accessible and user-friendly.

5.

MAPPING WITH MOUTH MERIDIANS

In traditional Chinese medicine (TCM), meridians are a network of energy channels through the body that distribute qi (life force or energy) but are imperceptible to most scientific methods of observation. Nonetheless, TCM credits meridians with performing a variety of tasks to maintain health and well-being. Each meridian is named for the organ it is most closely linked with, though meridian names should be understood as referring to energy systems rather than discreet anatomical organs which could be identified in a dissection.

Ten of these conceptual organs are categorized as either solid (zang) or hollow (fu). Heart, liver, spleen, lung and kidney are zang organs, and each is paired with a fu organ: small intestine, gall bladder, stomach, large intestine, and bladder. They are also characterized as yin or yang within the same pairs. Each pair of meridians is governed by one of five transformative elements or processes (wood, fire, earth, metal and water), which in turn are associated with emotions (qi qing).

There are four additional meridians: the overarching central and governing meridians; and the triple burner (aka san jiao) and pericardium (aka circulation-sex).

All these fourteen main tributaries of the meridian system are accessible inside your mouth. The meridian channels flow inside your cheeks and lips, and over the palates. They surface at meridian points in the mucus membranes of the mouth.

Every tooth is adjacent to a pair of energy channels, although there is a zone of four energy channels occupying a relatively large area at the very back of your mouth, closest to where wisdom teeth usually sit, and extending towards the joint connecting lower jaw to upper jaw. Each tooth is influenced by, and has influence on, the pair of meridians they come in contact with.

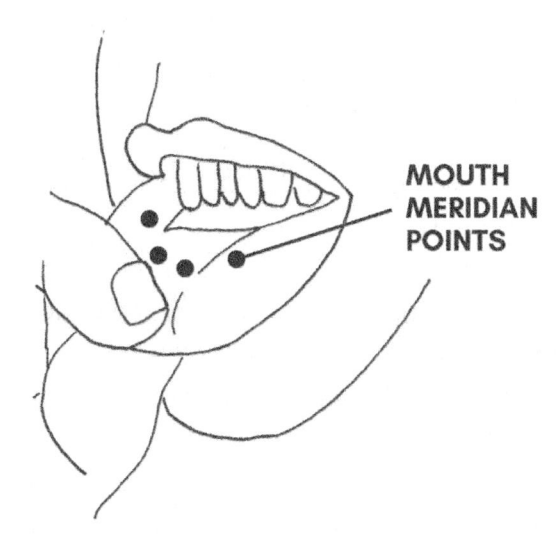

Location of kidney and bladder meridian points in the mouth

Meridians at the front of the mouth

Kidney and bladder meridians pass through the front of your mouth, at the interface between your inner world and the outer world. In TCM these two meridians belong to the water element, which represents peace. The strengths of the kidney and bladder meridians include patience and decisiveness, which are two different ways of creating a sense of safety in relation to external situations.

You can find these meridian points located on the inside of the lips near the central frenula, opposite the center of the central and lateral incisor teeth's standard positions (teeth 7, 8, 9, 10, 23, 24, 25, 26). They are also associated with the genitals (those other lips) and reproductive organs.

The bladder meridian can be vulnerable to fears arising from inner thoughts such as shame. Teeth and gums touching this meridian may become unbalanced by mildly fearful behaviors or patterns of timidity, shyness, cautiousness and superstition. It could be blocked by more debilitating fears such as anxiety, phobias or paranoia.

The teeth and gums adjacent to the kidney meridian are vulnerable to feeling helpless, listless, lethargic and deeply exhausted. This meridian can be unbalanced if your will is broken and you feel like nothing you do matters or could make a difference.

Meridians at the corner of your mouth

The liver and gallbladder meridians pass through the tightest curve of the jawbones' arch, between the front and side of your mouth. In TCM these meridians belong to the wood element, which represents contentment. Liver and gallbladder meridians thrive on taking responsibility with self-confidence and humbleness.

These meridian points are located on the inside of the lips opposite the center of each canine tooth's standard positions (teeth

6, 11, 22, 27). They are also associated with hips and knees, and the eyes.

The teeth and gums adjacent to the liver meridian are vulnerable to uncontrolled expressions of anger or outbursts of rage. The gallbladder meridian can get blocked with suppressed anger such as resentment and frustration. These meridians can get out of balance from internalizing patterns of helplessness or blaming others. Symptoms in this part of the mouth may get activated by excess pride, judging others or manipulative behaviour.

MERIDIANS DOWNHILL ON THE SIDE OF YOUR MOUTH

The lung and large intestine meridians cross over the inside of your cheeks from the upper premolars to the lower molars. In TCM these two meridians are associated with the metal element, which represents fulfillment. Their strengths include compassion and cheerfulness. They thrive with letting go of anything that doesn't support your highest good.

You'll find these meridian points located on the inside of the cheeks opposite the center of each of the top premolars and bottom molars' standard positions (teeth 4, 5, 12, 13, 18, 19, 30, 31).

The lung meridian is vulnerable to sadness in all its forms from melancholy to depression and chronic grief. It can become unbalanced by burdensome guilt, regret, apathy or powerlessness.

The large intestine meridian is sensitive to feeling uptight, dogmatic, compulsive or overcritical. The meridian may also fall out of balance by externalizing those feelings into intolerance, prejudice, contempt, or scornfulness.

MERIDIANS UPHILL ON THE SIDE OF YOUR MOUTH

The stomach and spleen meridians cross over the inside of your cheeks from the lower premolars to the upper molars. In TCM these two meridians are associated with the earth element, which represents confidence. Their strengths include harmony and satisfaction.

These meridian points are located on the inside of the cheeks adjacent to the center of each of the lower premolars and top molars' standard positions (teeth 4, 5, 12, 13, 18, 19, 30, 31).

The stomach meridian is vulnerable to disappointment, deprivation, hunger, or greed. This part of the mouth may absorb the emotional hurts of other people's criticism and unreliability, and suffer when you respond to them with disgust, doubt or bitterness.

The spleen meridian is vulnerable to overthinking and brooding in all forms including anxiety, alienation, cynicism, pensiveness and envy. It can be unbalanced by fear of forgetfulness, rejection and disapproval.

MERIDIANS AT THE BACK OF YOUR MOUTH

The heart, small intestine, triple warmer and pericardium meridians sit beside and behind the wisdom (teeth 1, 16, 17, 32). These meridians are all associated with the fire element, which represents joy. Their strengths include love, hope, openness, empathy, co-operation, appreciation, calmness, generosity and lightness. They thrive with mental clarity, decisiveness and romantic love.

The heart and small intestine meridian points are located on the inside of the cheeks opposite the center of each wisdom tooth's standard position. The triple warmer and pericardium meridian points sit behind wisdom teeth, in front of the TMJ joint connecting the upper and lower jaws.

The heart meridian is vulnerable to insecurity and can become unbalanced with agitation, mania and hysteria.

The small intestine meridian is vulnerable to feeling unappreciated or broken-hearted, leading to low self-worth and powerlessness or hatred and defensiveness. This part of the mouth can be blocked by feeling nervous, insecure, indecisive,

MAPPING WITH MOUTH MERIDIANS

self-doubting, hyper-vigilant or secretive.

The triple warmer meridian is vulnerable to despair, despondence, gloominess, heaviness, and hopelessness. It may be unbalanced by unwelcome solitude or extreme exhaustion.

The pericardium can become blocked by stubbornly holding onto the past, which can feel like humiliation, remorse, jealousy or inhibitions.

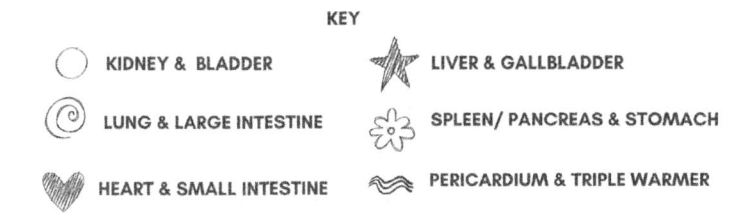

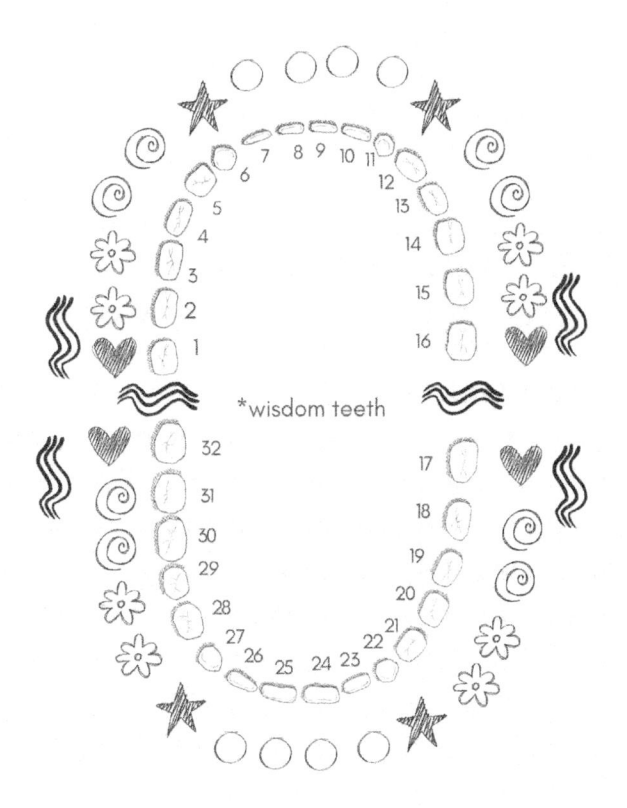

KEY

○ KIDNEY & BLADDER

✦ LIVER & GALLBLADDER

@ LUNG & LARGE INTESTINE

❀ SPLEEN/ PANCREAS & STOMACH

♥ HEART & SMALL INTESTINE

∿ PERICARDIUM & TRIPLE WARMER

*wisdom teeth

Mouth Meridians

6.

MAPPING QUADRANTS OF THE MOUTH

Metaphysically and anatomically, you can divide your mouth horizontally into upper and lower jaws; and vertically into right and left sides. Building on the mystical ground of mouth meridians, the themes expressed in each section of the mouth are infused with their own culture, like neighborhoods in a town.

UPPER JAW: ORIGINS

The upper jaw (maxilla) embodies social and emotional dynamics of relating to your family or culture of origin. Fused to the skull, the upper jaw expresses qualities of thoughtfulness, introspection, sensitivity, intuition and self-awareness.

Your upper jaw is associated with dreams and intentions and can be understood as a representation of where and how you visualize the future, set goals and make plans. Conversely, it can hold onto the ways you are influenced by your past, your ancestors and maybe even past lives.

The maxilla may represent your feelings about what you want

and wish for. Symptoms concentrated in your upper jaw may indicate a problem with recognizing or accepting your dreams. Perhaps there is a conflict between your background and your desires.

Lower jaw: Actions

The lower jaw (mandible) embodies the dynamics of your relationships with peers, partners and your own children. Connected to the upper jaw by robust joints and strong muscles, the lower jaw actively represents what you do and say. Your lower jaw can carry qualities of courage, authenticity and decisiveness.

Symptoms concentrated in your lower jaw may suggest you have held back from speaking out or taking action. Lower jaw symptoms may indicate regret for past choices or discomfort with current circumstances.

Left side: Private

The energy of the left side of your mouth tends to be associated with your inner thoughts, imagination, intuition, and private life with family, children, hobbies, creativity and leisure. It thrives when your family or home represents a place where you can rest and re-establish yourself to regain strength, where you find refuge from the world and can freely express your personal preferences.

Right side: Public

The right side of your mouth represents how you act towards other people who are outside of your family and intimate relationships. It reacts to dynamics of belonging and exclusion in the public sphere including work. Your right side can also embody conflicts with values or affiliations to cultural, religious, professional and community groups and leaders.

Front and back of the mouth

The front of your mouth is most closely associated with your more existential relationships, starting with your parents and your own body before moving back through intimate relationships with a spouse, lovers, colleagues, or closest friends. Further back in the mouth symptoms are more likely to reflect how you engage with the challenges of adult life including establishing a home and career or being a parent while the back molars and wisdom teeth tend to respond to more abstract issues such as politics, religion, values etc.

Quadrant themes

Upper left quadrant relates to your family of origin and your physical body. It is linked to common sense and instinctive thinking, the ideas that seem natural to you. It is sensitive to your self-image and the perceptions of the world that you learned from your family.

Upper right quadrant relates to society and your spiritual life. It is linked to the cerebral, logical thinking that enables you to function in groups outside of your closest family. It responds to social relationships, perceptions of family status and identities of cultural belonging. It is sensitive to your relationship with your higher self and inner consciousness.

Lower right quadrant relates to the community you join outside of your family. It responds to the state of your peer relationships with colleagues, teammates or friends in school, clubs or the workplace. It is sensitive to conflicts around competition, status and ambition.

Lower left quadrant relates to your home and your intimate relationships as an adult. It is linked to your sense of place. It can be vulnerable to any way that you lack a home with restorative, secure, nurturing qualities.

INTERPRETING SYMPTOMS ACROSS QUADRANTS

Dr Beyer notes that when symptoms appear symmetrically between right and left sides, or between upper and lower jaws metaphysical meanings carry more weight.

Symmetrical left-right symptoms may reflect how your professional life impacts your home life, and visa versa. Symmetrical upper-lower symptoms show how your adult life carries echoes of your childhood, family circumstances or ancestral trauma.

When your upper and lower molars aren't aligned enough to chew properly, it may represent a resistance or block to deeply engaging with life challenges, either in the past or as an ongoing pattern.

Your jaw skewing to right suggests that you might have avoided expressing emotions or been responding to difficulties in close relationships with too much emphasis on action over introspection. Alternatively, your jaw skewing to left may mean you have avoided economic responsibilities or not processed emotional blocks to pursuing your professional or academic ambitions.

7.

MAPPING TYPES OF TEETH

There are eight types of adult teeth, and each type shares developmental characteristics in common, in the same way that contemporary house designs are recognizable from street to street in a suburban development. Even when there are teeth missing (or extra), or they have moved out of alignment in your jaw, the metaphysical vernacular for each *type* of tooth stays true.

INCISORS IN FRONT: INFANT INFLUENCES

Open your mouth to speak or smile, to breathe deeply, or to eat or drink… and what do you see?

Orthodontists nicknamed the top and bottom front teeth the 'social eight' because they are the only teeth visible in most interactions. That's why incisors are generally the teeth that you'll feel most self-conscious about.

Your lower incisors are usually the very first teeth that anyone ever saw, followed by the matching upper incisors. The first person who noticed these teeth was probably a parent. We all have a father who provided our 'y' chromosomes and a mother who provided our mitochondrial DNA. However, the individuals who connect us with our genetic heritage may or may not be the same individuals who taught us their family's culture and how to survive in the dominant paradigms of the wider culture. Both genetic and social influence can be embodied in your teeth.

The incisors are energetically associated with the individuals who cared for you when you were young, whether biological parents, adoptive or step-parents, or other adults such as grandparents, aunts and uncles, close and influential neighbors or teachers, perhaps even much older siblings who looked after you a lot.

The people who raised us taught us what is expected of girls and boys, men and women. Most people grow up barely conscious of gender conditioning, but it can be a source of terrible pain if those expectations don't fit your sense of self. You should always feel free to apply any of the gendered interpretations in this book as broadly as needed.

Existing metaphysical frameworks associate the right side with your father, other influential men and masculinity, and the left side with your mother, influential women and femininity. In these chapters I do my best to convey the meanings of teeth without using gendered stereotypes as shortcuts.

I believe the energetic meanings of teeth do not necessarily align with your sex or gender identity, or that of anyone else. The symptoms on your right and left side can mean different things according to your experiences of gender identity and sexuality.

In working with the metaphysical messages in your incisors and other teeth, any mention of Mother or Father can, and often should, be understood as archetypes rather than actual individual family members. It's not unusual for a caring adult who didn't conform with gender-assigned parenting roles to influence the opposite tooth.

The Mother archetype can be represented by the person you

received (or expected to receive) the most nurturing acceptance from while you were young. A Father archetype can be represented by the person who offered (or was expected to offer) an interface with the outside world, in the form of protection, boundaries and resources.

When you are trying to understand symptoms in your front teeth it's worth exploring any absence or inadequacy in the way you experienced the Mother and Father archetypes in your infancy or early childhood. The purpose is not to assign blame but to better understand what beliefs or behaviors you may have internalized and embodied in your mouth.

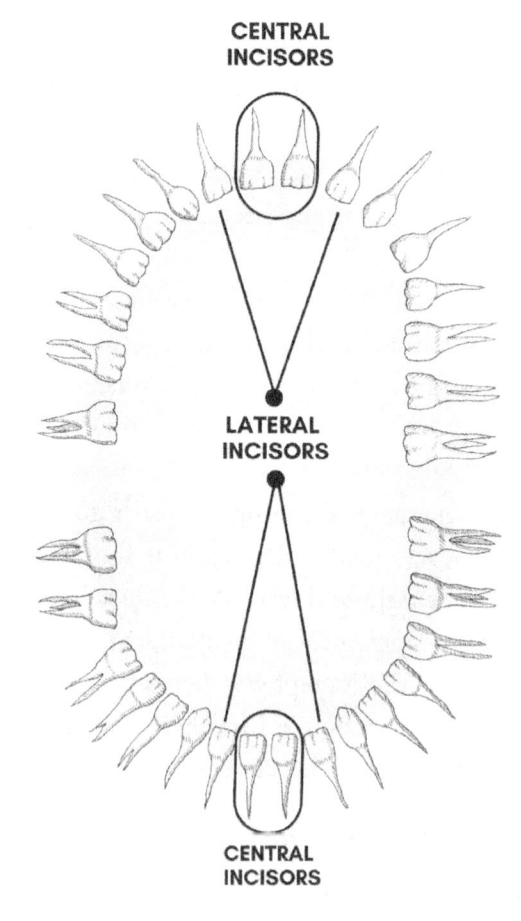

Central and lateral incisor tooth types

Central incisors: Socialization

Central incisors (9, 8, 24, 25) are the first teeth that appear in a baby's mouth from around six months old, the first teeth to fall out around six years old and the first adult teeth to grow in soon after that.

These teeth hold the energy of your relationships to the individuals who cared for you as an infant, or from pseudo parent-child dynamics echoed in later relationships with a boss, teacher, coach or therapist. Wherever these current or recent influences seem relevant, you are also likely to encounter insights about infancy and childhood and the dynamics of your family back then, as you become more attuned to the messages from these teeth.

Your upper central incisors represent how you learned what was required to be accepted in your family and wider communities, especially other people's perceptions of you as a boy or girl growing into a man or a woman.

Your lower central incisors represent how you received and responded to those social expectations, especially of femininity and masculinity, as they were projected onto you from birth.

Folk beliefs about central incisors include: a gap between the top central incisors indicates that your parents experienced separate lives from each other even if they were living together; and when both right central incisors (25 and 8) are jutting forward in front of the left central incisors (24 and 9) it indicates a violent and domineering father in your family.

Dr Caffin links the right central incisors with the astrological sign of Leo and its ruling luminary the Sun, the Kabbalistic meaning of the Hebrew letter י (yod) and the element hydrogen. She links the left central incisors with the astrological sign of Aquarius and its ruling planet Uranus, the Kabbalistic meaning of the Hebrew letter ם (final mem) and the element oxygen. She also identifies the central incisors with symbolic animals: the narwhal and the unicorn.

Lateral incisors: Internalization

Lateral incisors (10, 7, 26, 23) usually appear in your mouth soon after the central incisors show up on the top and bottom jaws, first as baby teeth, then again when those fall out and are replaced with adult teeth.

Lateral incisors represent how you internalized the qualities of the archetypes of their adjacent central incisors. They can hold your feelings about, and be vulnerable to disputes with, your parents (or parent figures) in relation to what they taught about how to belong in your family or community.

Your upper lateral incisors represent both the conscious rules of survival that you defined for yourself from childhood onwards, and your unconscious habitual compliance with the cultural norms of the place you grew up. When these upper laterals protrude it may embody how you resisted and rebelled against your parents. Receding upper lateral incisors may indicate a lack of independent thought or action (Caffin).

Your lower lateral incisors represent adult roles you tried to conform with because of those internalized expectations. When these lower laterals protrude, they may embody how you established yourself independent of your family's influence. Receding lower lateral incisors may represent the effects of complying with family expectations that aren't aligned with your true self or highest good.

Caffin links the right lateral incisors with the astrological sign of Capricorn and its ruling planet Saturn; the Kabbalistic meaning of the Hebrew letter ב (beth) and the element aluminum. She links left lateral incisors with the astrological sign of Cancer and its ruling luminary the Moon; the Kabbalistic meaning of the Hebrew letter ף (final phe) and the element phosphorus. She identifies lateral incisors symbolically with the cow and the elephant.

Canines: Power dynamics

Canine teeth (6, 11, 22, 27) have more alternative names in English than any other type of tooth: cuspid, eye teeth or vampire fangs, so called for their unique, slightly extended and pointed tip. The canines are singletons (like wisdom teeth) in each quadrant dominated by pairs of incisors, premolars and molars. While the pairs of teeth are associated with particular life stages, the canines represent different kinds of power relationships.

Baby canines usually appear between 16 and 20 months of age, just as you are learning to speak. The permanent (adult) canines usually first erupt in the lower jaw around 9 years old, while the upper canines arrive around 11 or 12 years of age.

Beyer believes that canines are linked to the language areas of the brain that were developing as those teeth emerged. They embody the importance of language for defining your place in society throughout your life.

Canine teeth can be influenced by power dynamics in your relationships. In the upper jaw they are associated with your family or culture of origin. In the lower jaw they represent the partnerships, groups and households you join or create as an adult.

Canine teeth thrive with the kinds of creativity and pleasure that flourish within limits. They can be made vulnerable when there's change, movement and growth without conscious structure or deliberate direction.

Caffin links the right canine teeth with the astrological sign of Gemini and its ruling planet Mars, the Kabbalistic meaning of the Hebrew letter צ (tsadi) and the mineral carbon. She links the left canine teeth with the astrological sign of Taurus and its ruling planet Venus; the Kabbalistic meaning of the Hebrew letter ר (resh) and the mineral nitrogen. She names the deer and the giraffe as symbolic animals for canine teeth.

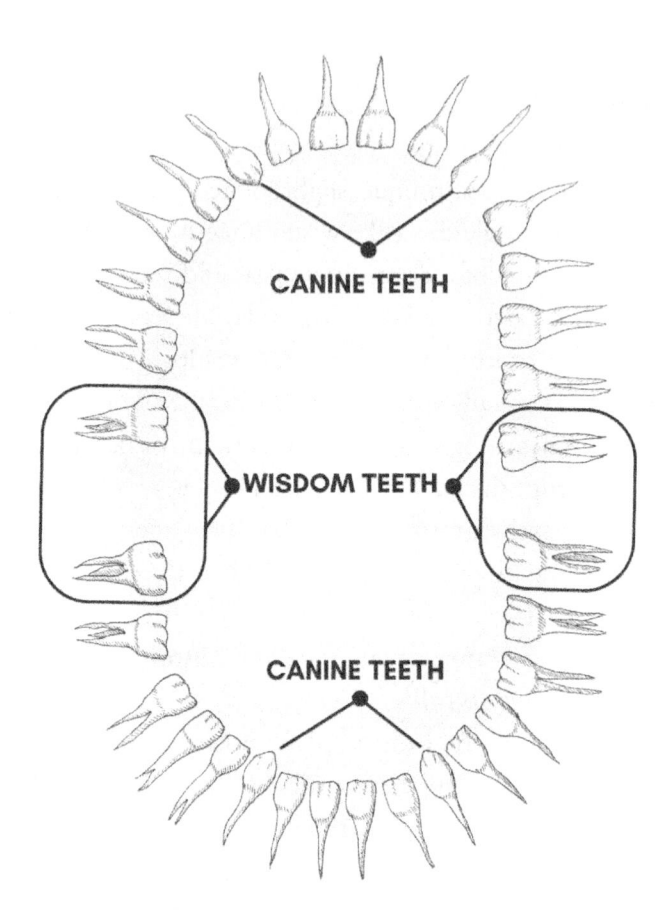

Canine and wisdom tooth types

Premolar teeth: Establishing identity

Premolars erupt after the baby molars fall out, usually between 9 and 12 years old. Their growth coincides with the stage of brain development associated with the ego, identity and sense of self.

The baby molars leave behind a space for the adult premolars that has been shaped by what your earliest experiences taught you about being an individual in relationship with others. As a very young child, when your survival depended entirely on other people, you learned what you needed to do, or not do, in order to get your needs met.

Premolars are sensitive to emotionally charged but unconscious memories of the life stages when you were first learning how to fit into family and friendships. These teeth can hold energies of security and survival, belonging and exclusion, promises and betrayals.

Caffin identifies the lion and the wolf as symbolic animals associated with premolar teeth.

First premolars: Intimacy

The first premolars (5, 12, 21, 28) embody your emotional or instinctive responses to your immediate environment and the people closest to you. They can pick up on the way your sense of self is established by expressing your likes and dislikes. Your preferences and pleasures are points of connection with some people yet can distance you from others.

It's common practice for orthodontists to extract young teenagers' first premolars in preparation for installing braces in a crowded jaw. A standardized smile is not the only compromise to individuality to result from this widespread orthodontic intervention.

Losing any of your premolars may make it feel difficult to say (or even know) what you want or think. You might prefer to go along with the group, or to follow a strong leader, rather than act independently. You may even struggle to identify what gives you pleasure.

Caffin links the first premolar teeth with the astrological sign of Aries and its ruling planet Mars, the Kabbalistic meaning of the Hebrew letter ו (vav) and the mineral silica.

Second premolars: Support

The second premolars (4, 13, 20, 29) reflect how you relate to the things you do or make for pleasure: your creativity and hobbies.

These teeth reflect relationships in which dynamics are overtly changing, such as between parents and rapidly developing children (you're the child in relation to upper teeth, and the adult in the relation to lower teeth). Second premolars are sensitive to feeling guilty or ashamed, especially about not fulfilling your potential, being authentic or being loyal.

They draw your attention to where you don't feel worthy of pleasure or ease in your life. These feelings can be traced back to lack of attachment and safety when you were a child because that's when you would have absorbed the idea of not deserving.

Caffin links second premolars with the astrological sign of Libra and its ruling planet Venus; the Kabbalistic meaning of the Hebrew letter שׁ (shin) and the mineral calcium.

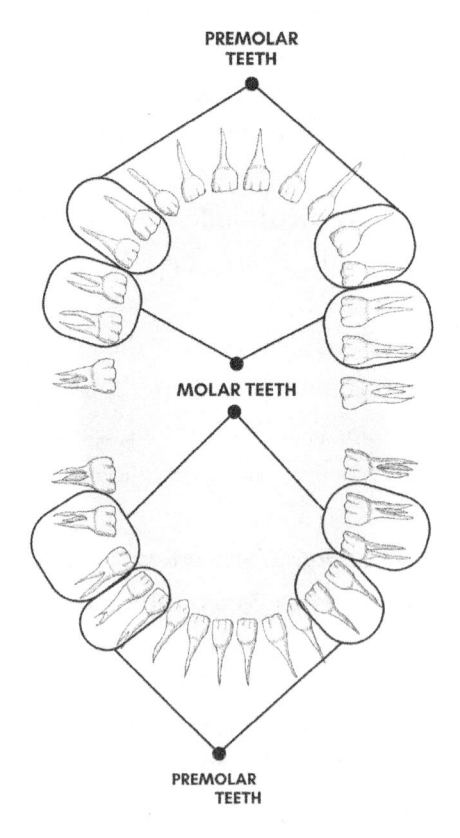

Premolar and molar tooth types

Molars: Adulthood's challenges

The further back in your mouth we venture, the more your teeth are influenced by the autonomy of your teenage and adult life than the upbringing of your childhood.

The three permanent molars (wisdom teeth are third molars) in each quadrant originated as a single germ in the embryo. Adult molars developed underneath the baby molars while your capacity to use language to meet your emotional, spiritual and psychological needs was developing in your frontal cortex. Baby molars are impacted by a child's need to differentiate themselves from their parents (Beyer).

Your first adult molar typically erupted through your gum at around 6 years old, at the same time as most children are developing more emotional and social autonomy from your family. Anecdotally, some primary (elementary) school teachers believe that the abstract thinking required for reading and arithmetic come much easier for children once their first molars are visible.

The second molar typically erupted when you were about 12 years old, at the time when your brain was developing the capacity for even more independent thinking. There is some evidence that both first and second adult molars can erupt earlier than usual when there has been stress in early childhood (Cassidy et al).

Caffin links molars with the astrological sign of Gemini and its ruling planet Mercury; the Kabbalistic meaning of the Hebrew letter ה (he); the mineral sulfur and mythical animals, the centaur (first molars) and Pegasus (second molars).

First molars: Status

The first molars (3, 14, 19, 30) reflect your status in different domains. They erupt around six years of age, when many children start to establish independent relationships outside of their immediate family's influence. That's around the stage of becoming conscious that you can be perceived as one kind of person in the classroom, another in private with friends and both those roles may be different from how you are treated by your caregivers.

First molars are sensitive to challenges of code switching: changing your language and behaviour in different contexts. These teeth can embody the feeling of not fitting in, especially if you don't have at least one domain in your life where you can relax and show your full, authentic, true self.

Second molars: Authenticity

Second molars (2, 15, 18, 31) erupt in the mouth around twelve years of age when hormones are awakening to herald puberty. From this age you have access to more reflective consciousness and a more sophisticated concept of time.

The second molar is associated with the developmental tasks of adolescence when you ricochet between extremes of acknowledging your unique thoughts and individual identity, and feeling a strong impulse to fit in and belong with your people. You may be concerned with creating or joining a new group of friends who share your perspectives. Or you may withhold your point of view in order to maintain membership in a group you belong to but are starting to think differently from.

Second molars signal access to autonomous thought: the ability to think for yourself. But thinking differently from your group can create conflict and threaten your sense of belonging, so that this experience may be reflected in the health of second molars.

Wisdom teeth: Codification

Wisdom teeth (1, 16, 17, 32) connect you with the collective culture of your ancestral lineage.

Wisdom teeth are the last new teeth that most people will ever see emerge. They most commonly appear around 17–25 years old although it is not unusual to have wisdom teeth erupt in your thirties, forties or even later.

The arrival of wisdom teeth can represent your readiness to step into a new developmental stage of adult life and personal growth. The collective influences on these teeth can mean that your wisdoms come through at the same time as a cohort of your age group who are each on their own profound spiritual journey. When I see several of my adult clients present with similar wisdom symptoms and stories within a few weeks of each other, it suggests that there are collective energy shifts pulling this group into the next stage of their soul development.

Wisdom teeth below the surface of the gum are described as impacted. The longer a wisdom tooth stays impacted the more likely it is to cause problems including crowding other teeth, causing infection, decay or cavities. Many people experience impacted wisdom teeth that grow at an odd angle, often butting into the next tooth and crowding the whole row of teeth or pushing their bite out of alignment.

Wisdom teeth that stay below the gums into your twenties or beyond, especially if they are causing discomfort or disease, may metaphysically represent your resistance to the next stage of development or maturity.

If partially impacted wisdoms rise and fall in your gums repeatedly – putting you at risk of infection if any food particles or bacterial film is carried back into the gum – this may represent feeling ambivalence, rather than full-blown resistance, towards adult responsibilities.

About twenty percent of people never develop a full set of four wisdom teeth buds, which is thought to be an evolutionary response to modern human jaws getting smaller and narrower than those of our ancestors. Metaphysically, it may also be a collective evolutionary response to the expansion of literacy and the availability of information from other sources than oral traditions. Individually, not growing wisdom teeth may indicate a capacity to easily adapt to the rapidly shifting energies of contemporary life.

When wisdom teeth are missing for any reason you can compensate energetically by engaging with sources and systems of wisdom to expand your social awareness and be more consciously inclusive of other ways of thinking.

Caffin links wisdom teeth with the astrological planet Saturn, the Kabbalistic meaning of the Hebrew letter ת (tav), the mineral magnesium and fish as a symbol.

8.

MAPPING TOOTH SURFACES

Dentists routinely make note of the particular surface of the tooth where a cavity is located using descriptors such as labial or lingual. Dr Beyer has identified unique metaphysical associations for cavities that develop on different surfaces. Zooming into such close focus within the metaphorical neighborhood of your mouth is like describing individual rooms inside of a thoroughly lived-in house. Although any bedroom can be recognized as a bedroom, every room (surface) in every house (tooth) is distinctive because of the unique personality of its occupant.

Labial and **buccal** surfaces are outward facing. The surfaces of the front teeth that touch the inside of your lips are called labial. Further back in the mouth, the surfaces that touch the inside of your cheeks are called buccal. Beyer gives a relational association to these outward-facing surfaces. Depending on the particular tooth, these surfaces can reflect how you present yourself to the world, or how others perceive you. Decay or other symptoms on these surfaces may be trying to draw your attention to conflicts with other people.

Lingual surfaces touch the tongue. Beyer gives these inward-facing surfaces introspective associations. They can reflect your private thoughts and feelings and may be vulnerable to self-criticism or self-harming behaviors. Cavities or other symptoms on these surfaces could point to unhealthy secrets, private disappointments, or unfulfilled desires.

Mesial surfaces are in between teeth, on the side of the tooth oriented towards either the front or center line of the body (depending on tooth placement). In Beyer's framework they are associated with witnessing. Mesial surfaces may represent how you observe the adjacent tooth's archetype, so that between-teeth cavities may be embodying resentment, intolerance or responsibility towards an individual or group represented by the adjacent tooth.

Distal refers to surfaces that are in between teeth and oriented towards the back of the jaw (away from the front and center). Beyer associates them with feeling stuck. Distal surfaces can reflect your unresolved conflicts with an individual or group represented by the adjacent tooth's archetype, so that between-teeth cavities may be telling a story of judgment or blame.

Cervical refers to the part of the tooth that is closest to the gumline, and Beyer attributes different associations depending on which side of the tooth is affected. Decay on the outward-facing gumline may reflect a tension between action and self-control. The symptoms on the tongue-facing gumline may embody an oppressive silence with a life or death quality.

Mapping Tooth Surfaces

Apex and **occlusal** surfaces are the hardest working part of any tooth. Apex refers to the sharp edge of the front teeth that is used for biting. Occlusal refers to the flat chewing surface of the back teeth (which isn't really flat but rough with cusps, troughs and ridges). For Beyer, caries or other symptoms on these surfaces may have an association with feeling abandoned, forgotten or betrayed.

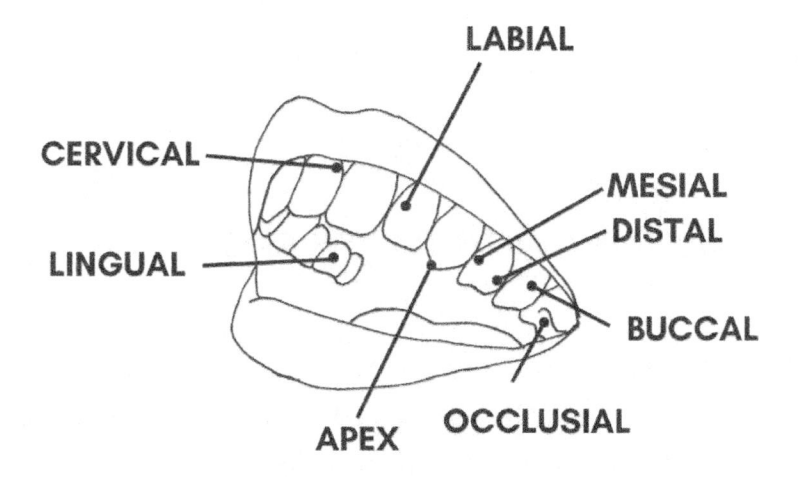

Tooth surfaces

9.

MAPPING WITH TOOTH ARCHETYPES

This chapter details the Tooth Archetypes framework I have developed over years of working holistically with oral health issues for myself and with coaching clients. Through this work I have identified a distinct archetype or personality for each of the 32 teeth, as outlined below.

MEET YOUR CENTRAL INCISOR ARCHETYPES

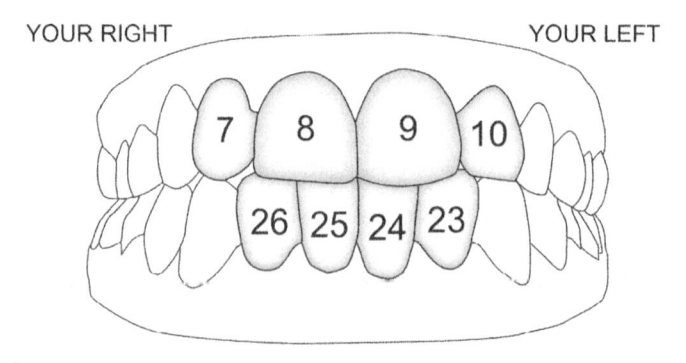

Identifying your central and lateral incisor teeth

Nurturer archetype:
Upper left central incisor (9)

The Nurturer tooth reflects your relationship with your mother or anyone who occupies a significant nurturing role in your life. It may hold the memories of your first experiences of being held and cared for as an infant. It not only embodies the quality of connection you've had (or not) with your own mother but it is also influenced by your relationships with matriarchal figures, your family of origin in general, and your own body.

The strength of this tooth lies with taking time to be restored, nourished, rested, reset and protected wherever you go, or whatever you do. It thrives when you follow your intuition and trust your desires.

This tooth is vulnerable to estrangement from your mother (or a mother figure), particularly when there was conflict about your body (e.g. food, clothing or sexuality); or an estrangement between your mother and father. It's also vulnerable to self-denial or homelessness.

Difficulties with fertility, sterility or impotence may affect this tooth. Symptoms can embody a hidden self-hatred, which undermines your good intentions for a healthy lifestyle, perhaps even feeling as though you wish you'd never been born.

Symptoms may also develop on the Nurturer tooth if your self-image seems incompatible with your physical body, for instance if you wanted to be a dancer but were rejected from professional opportunities because of your body shape. It can hold shame or other hurts related to body dysmorphia or misgendering.

Tooth 9 may store individual or collective trauma from dehumanizing experiences such as colonialism, racism, classism, ablism or homophobia. It could carry unconscious ancestral guilt for communications that led to others losing their land, resources or quality of life, particularly if your heritage connects you with colonizers or invaders. Or the tooth may hold memories of being unable to defend yourself when judged unfairly.

When this tooth is asking for attention
- Try tuning into your somatic awareness while thinking about how you were caring for your body in the weeks or months before the symptoms started.
- What are the physical sensations you can feel, what do they mean and how can you respond appropriately?
- Sleep when you are tired, eat when you are hungry, drink when you are thirsty.
- Consider whether you have a tendency to use stubborn silence as a form of self-harm.

Leader archetype: Upper right central incisor (8)

The Leader tooth reflects your relationship with your father or anyone with a significant protective role in your life, including patriarchal figures or leaders. It embodies the quality of connection you've had (or not) with your own father or it may hold onto your youthful perception of the relationship between your mother and father.

Alternatively, this tooth could be influenced by conflicts with any dominant individual in a role which included setting limits and rules that you were expected to obey, or a responsibility to protect you, such as a teacher, coach or boss.

The strength of this tooth lies in getting inspired with a project, making a plan to realize it and having the momentum to carry out that objective.

This tooth is vulnerable to a lack of willpower, feelings of helplessness or being overwhelmed, or shame for not achieving your goals.

This tooth can hold memories (your own or ancestral) of

conflict or tension in a parasocial or impersonal relationship such as with a cult leader, a CEO, a president or the Pope. It could even embody your concept of God-the-Father or the patriarchy as an influential force in your life.

Symptoms may reflect a fear (or reality) of sanctions or deprivation from choosing autonomy over compliance, rejecting societal expectations or having conflict with authority figures.

When this tooth is asking for attention
- Look at what was going on with your professional goals or public aspirations in the months or weeks before the symptoms started.
- Were you pushing yourself too hard, taking on extra work or failing to set boundaries with your employer?
- Consider whether you believe you need to change yourself to fulfill your potential or you are censoring yourself to comply with outer expectations.

Beast archetype:
Lower right central incisor (25)

The Beast tooth embodies your intentions to be competent, for example by taking action towards educational, professional or status goals.

This tooth holds the energy of forward momentum and doing whatever it takes to survive, but also the energy of frustrated tantrums when your will is blocked. Think of the toddler who wants to zip up their own coat without help, despite not having the fine motor skills required, so they end up thrashing around on the floor, screaming.

This tooth is supported by reasonable self-confidence and valid self-belief. It thrives when you pursue meaningful goals effectively, especially as you become more skilled through your own efforts.

This tooth may embody fears that your shadow self is dark and dominant. It is vulnerable when you react to frustrating situations with suppressed anger or conversely, with unregulated rage and aggression. Symptoms may reflect a belief that you are entitled to success without effort, or a habit of blaming others for your own lack of competence.

Tooth 25 can hold memories (your own or ancestral) of a being raised by a violent, strict parent figure who did not tolerate failure and who both provoked your anger and punished its expression. It may carry personal or generational trauma from being bullied, marginalized or mocked.

When the tooth is prominent in front of adjacent teeth it indicates you may have a pattern of responding to the challenges of adult life with too much aggression.

When the tooth recedes behinds adjacent teeth it indicates that you may react to difficulties with a facade of passiveness or niceness that conceals suppressed anger.

When this tooth is asking for attention
- Look for where you feel frustrated about not achieving your goals at the speed, or in the way, that you want.
- Is your inner voice harsh and cruel?
- Do you fear that your temper could flare out of control?
- Consider whether you've lost perspective regarding the appropriate expression of righteous anger.

Doll archetype:
Lower left central incisor (24)

The Doll tooth embodies a willingness to passively accept the expectations and projections of a powerful, overbearing or inconsiderate parent or partner. Issues in this tooth may represent a pattern of people pleasing, or reflect situations where you accepted domination, or endured deprivation, in order to survive.

It can hold energies of emotional vulnerability, fragility and weakness or a desire to be protected and supported. Think of the toddler who hides shyly behind their parent's legs. The flip side of its energy is feeling like you'd rather die than depend on someone else.

The strength of this tooth lies in patience, tolerance, self-reflection and receptivity. It thrives with your ability to understand other people's emotional state and respond in ways that meet your own needs as well as theirs.

This tooth is vulnerable to performing a docile or disassociated version of femininity, but also to acting with passive-aggressive manipulation, sulks, silent treatment or self-harm.

This tooth can hold memories (your own or ancestral) of manipulation and exploitation, rape or abuse, or of being economically and emotionally dependent on a more powerful person. It can embody numbing out impassively to cope with abusive language or to avoid confrontation with a person in power.

When this tooth is asking for attention
- Look at the power imbalances in your intimate relationships, such as where you give too much without receiving anything in return.
- Explore where it feels safer to go along with others' expectations than assert your own autonomy.
- Do you need to figure out or speak up about what *you* really want in family or intimate relationships?
- Consider where you fear showing vulnerability.

Meet your lateral incisor archetypes

Priestess archetype:
Upper left lateral incisor (10)

The Priestess tooth represents the habits and norms of caring for your own body that you learned from your primary caregiver. This tooth represents the archetype of Mother-as-Healer: an ideal reliable, consistent source of nourishment, safety and restoration.

It holds your understanding of what is required to care for your own wellbeing and has an energetic connection to your general health.

The strength of this tooth lies in mindfully following traditions and rituals to care for yourself and others, such as consistent daily practices or alignment with lunar cycles. This tooth also thrives with self-love and intuitive self-care guided by your own pleasure.

The Priestess tooth is vulnerable to health advice or fad diets that undermine your own somatic body-awareness. It can embody long-term conflicts with a mother figure about food, hygiene or clothing. It may respond to feeling isolated because you are unable to express your inner truths clearly or because you feel contempt towards the people around you for perceived differences in your morals or personal or domestic habits.

Tooth 10 can hold memories (your own or ancestral) of practicing physical self-denial, self-harm, or of body dysmorphia. It may carry collective trauma of being separated from cultural traditions of health and nourishment by colonialism, urbanization or immigration; or of living in a place or time when speaking your own language was forbidden or impossible. It may represent memories of being forced to change your self-care habits in order to be accepted after moving (or marrying) into a different culture or class.

When this tooth is asking for attention
- Look to your habitual ways of responding to your body's basic needs, what you learned as a child and your practices in the weeks or months before becoming aware of symptoms.
- Do you have a disproportionate fear of illness?
- Are you secretly ashamed of how you feed, clean, exercise or dress your own body?
- Consider reclaiming cultural or family practices around meals, hygiene, sleep etc.

Inner Critic archetype: Upper right lateral incisor (7)

The Inner Critic tooth embodies how you responded to harsh criticism from an authority figure such as a parent, boss or teacher. It can represent your ability and determination to articulate deeply held thoughts clearly and to argue for your own point of view confidently.

It may hold the energy of internalized patriarchal, colonial, or cultural expectations around work and status.

The strength of this tooth lies in compassionate self-awareness and an ability to give yourself constructive criticism as well as genuine self-appreciation. This tooth thrives when you can calmly observe your own thoughts and reflect on your emotions or actions to find inner conviction in the face of opposition. Connection with your authentic and unique identity, and confidence in your ability to articulate your true self clearly in public both support this tooth.

This tooth is vulnerable to harsh self-judgment and unreasonable expectations of yourself. It suffers when you berate yourself for making a mistake or have a pattern of never feeling good enough. It can embody rebellious thoughts that you never speak aloud or a desire for change that you never act upon. It can be undermined by feeling lost in the crowd because you lack individuality.

The Inner Critic tooth can hold memories (your own or ancestral) of being persecuted, punished or rejected for transgressing family rules or social norms. It may carry shame about non-conformity with gendered expectations.

When this tooth didn't develop due to absence of the tooth germ (perhaps with a cleft lip or palate) it may indicate there was a tyrant in the family who did not allow confrontation or opposition but who was nonetheless respected as a hero.

When this tooth is asking for attention
- Look for where you have internalized rules, roles, expectations or sanctions that don't support your highest good.
- Explore why you judge yourself so harshly or rebel against authority.
- Do you experience inner conflict about expressing yourself authentically?
- Consider whether breaking your own rules makes you feel more alive?

Guardian archetype:
Lower right lateral incisor (26)

The Guardian tooth relates to the security of your personal boundaries as you engage with the world beyond your home and intimate relationships.

It carries an energy of protection that can sometimes feel like restriction or imprisonment.

The strength of this tooth lies in safety, self-protection, saying no, and articulating energetic boundaries for work-life balance. It thrives when you stand up for yourself successfully.

This tooth is vulnerable to pushing good people away because you don't trust that you can keep yourself safe. Symptoms can be activated by a tendency to stay small, quiet and introverted for fear of being overridden. It can carry a feeling that you can't be trusted to take leadership, you are 'too much' or your aspirations are dangerous.

This tooth may hold memories of a complicated relationship with a parent who taught you how to defend yourself or alternatively a parent who failed to be protective. It can carry ancestral trauma from immigrating to a hostile environment where it seemed like survival depended on rigid mistrust.

When this tooth is asking for attention
- Check whether your paid work, activism or a friendship asks too much to the detriment of your personal life, especially in the weeks or months before your symptoms appeared.
- Do you find it hard to say no or find yourself easily persuaded by other people's strong opinions?
- Do you keep so silent that no one knows anything about you?
- Consider new ways to risk opening your heart without reckless disregard for safety.

Martyr archetype: Lower left lateral incisor (23)

The Martyr tooth relates to your role in intimate relationships as an adult, such as with a spouse, lover, live-in in-laws or your closest friend. It may also carry the residue of relationships with your closest family from when you were a child.

It can embody vulnerability, victimization, and self-sacrifice.

The strength of this tooth lies in feeling safe to open your heart and tolerate well-intentioned, but possibly clumsy, connections with the people closest to you. It thrives when your relationships are mutually beneficial and satisfying.

This tooth is vulnerable to being exploited, martyred or manipulated. Symptoms in this tooth can be activated by powerlessness or self-sacrifice. It can embody a feeling that your body betrays your mind or thinking that you don't deserve the kind of relationship you really want, or perhaps questioning whether you should keep on living.

Beyer describes how this tooth can hold memories (your own or ancestral) of losing privacy by renting out rooms, serving clients or running a restaurant in your home. It can hold collective trauma from living in occupied territory or personal trauma from losing power or property through marriage.

When this tooth is asking for attention
- Look at your energetic and physical boundaries or limits.
- Do you avoid confrontation at the expense of your well-being?
- Consider seeking help to recognize and address red flags in your relationships.
- Have you let yourself be taken advantage of or fooled?

Meet your canine archetypes

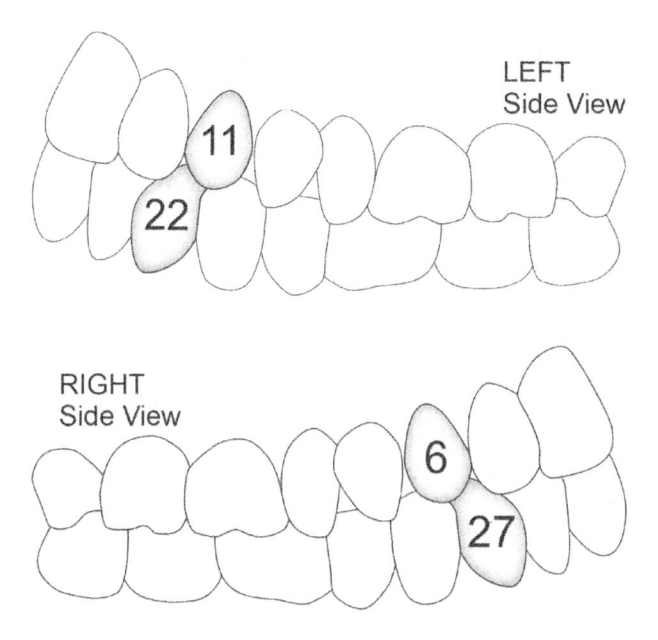

Identifying your canine teeth

Submission archetype: Upper left canine (11)

The Submission tooth responds to close relationships involving overt power dynamics in which you feel bound by duty, obedience or moral obligation.

The strength of this tooth lies in honest, healthy open negotiation and mutually agreed expectations.

This tooth is vulnerable to feeling powerless, violated or devalued; or experiencing deceit, cheating or catfishing.

Symptoms can also be activated by secondary trauma from witnessing someone else suffering deliberate cruelty.

This tooth can hold memories (your own or ancestral) of experiencing abuse, exploitation, manipulation, servitude, slavery or torture.

Beyer associates decay on the mesial surface of Submission

that touches the adjacent lateral incisor with relentless domestic responsibilities that straddle the line between family and employee. This could come from your own experience or an ancestor who suffered in such a role, for example, as a housekeeper who was also a mistress, a maiden aunt who was also a governess, an older sister who was also a babysitter, or an exploited live-in servant or slave.

When this tooth is asking for attention
- Look for where you need a break from other people's demands, or where you feel victimized, especially in the period leading up to symptoms appearing.
- Consider whether you are disproportionally distressed by a mundane memory that conceals an older, denser experience that needs to be brought into the light (such as a vow or curse)?
- What can you do to create calm flexible time management and peaceful tranquility in your home and family?

Commander archetype: Upper right canine (6)

The Commander tooth represents your response to external expectations. It can embody feelings about authority figures, institutions or your place in a hierarchy.

It holds the power of law and duty, both personally and professionally. It can reflect your relationship with an individual leader, a political movement or an organisation (such as the military).

The strength of this tooth lies in speaking truth to power, articulating yourself with powerful authority, or effectively expressing expectations that align with your authentic identity.

This tooth is vulnerable to any abuse of power, systemic mistreatment or feeling yourself the victim of unfair rules. It may reflect inner or outer conflicts in relation to laws, duties or obligations.

Symptoms may be activated if you make a commitment that goes against your values or your own better judgment.

This tooth can hold memories (your own or ancestral) of war, invasion or occupation. It can carry the burden of feeling persecuted and disorientated when being legally sanctioned or feeling helpless at the mercy of a dominant power.

When this tooth is asking for attention
- Consider how you react to commands and spoken expectations.
- When do you need to speak up for yourself with an authority figure?
- This tooth may need you to forgive yourself for guilt about following orders or abusing your power.

Collaborator archetype: Lower right canine (27)

The Collaborator tooth embodies professional or community relationships in which you contribute your time and energy to furthering a group project, a corporate mission or a collective movement.

It relates to situations in which you participate in the public sphere.

The strength of this tooth lies in helping, contributing and co-operating. It thrives when you can be patient while trying something new with a group and don't fear making mistakes in front of other people.

This tooth is vulnerable to intolerance, conflict and cancel culture. Symptoms may be activated when you are afraid of speaking or acting spontaneously.

This tooth can hold memories (your own or ancestral) of being rejected, kicked out, or disowned, perhaps by an unreasonably harsh family member or because of a professional conflict with a parent figure.

It may carry personal or collective trauma from humiliation or degradation associated with fighting with an army, collaborating with an enemy, or committing war crimes.

When this tooth is asking for attention
- Look for professional regrets or public mistakes in your past.
- Do you feel powerless to prevent a threat to the security of yourself, family or friends?
- Is there anything about which you feel rigidly judgmental?
- Do you tend to procrastinate for fear of making a mistake?

Servant archetype:
Lower left canine (22)

The Servant tooth represents a pattern of making yourself useful to earn acceptance in your family or another group in which you want to belong. It holds the energy of ongoing service, servitude, self-sacrifice and exploitation.

The strength of this tooth lies in feeling recognized and appreciated for your contributions. It thrives when you feel able take time for fun, meditation, exercise or creativity, and when your circumstances allow you to dream, grow and change.

It may carry memories (your own or ancestral) of sacrificing hopes and dreams to care for family members, working on the family farm or running the family business.

This tooth is vulnerable to feeling overwhelmed by the responsibilities of caring for many children or to staying in an oppressive marriage because of financial dependence.

This tooth may hold collective trauma from slavery, indentured service or exploitative domestic work.

When this tooth is asking for attention
- Look for where you put your needs last because you have to care for others.
- Do you feel trapped in a relationship or fear that leaving your current circumstances would mean you losing everything, and you won't be able to find another job, home or partner?
- Experiment with ways you can delegate or share your daily responsibilities.
- Explore options for radically changing your life.

MEET YOUR FIRST PREMOLAR ARCHETYPES

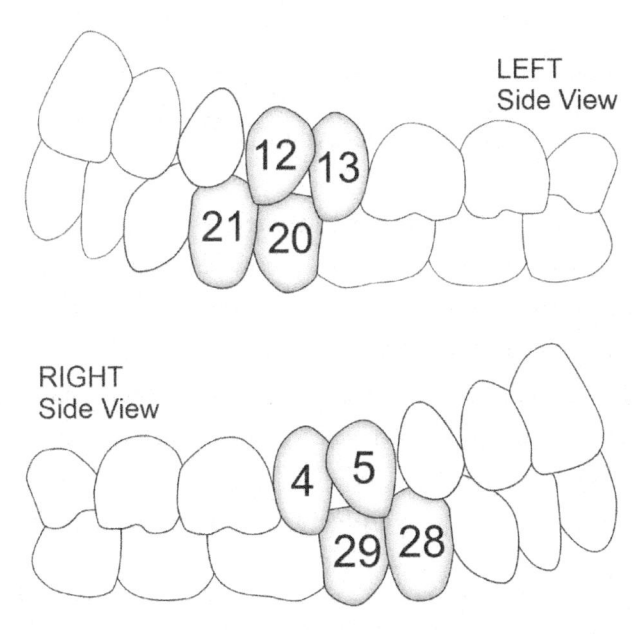

Identifying your premolar teeth

Forgiveness archetype:
Upper left first premolar (12)

The Forgiveness tooth represents desire for unconditional love and indulgence, a maternal kind of abundant love that eases your pain and allows you to recover after a disappointment or failure.

It holds energies of forgiveness, longing and relief.

The strength of this tooth lies in generously meeting your own needs and expressing your feelings with those closest to you.

Symptoms may be in response to feelings of guilt, self-denial, being starved for touch, fear of being yelled at, or of your own angry inner voice. It can carry a fear of abandonment and rejection, that makes it difficult for you to receive warm, loving affection.

This tooth can hold memories (your own or ancestral) of moving somewhere that, or with someone who, didn't observe or respect your family traditions. It is vulnerable to conflict with a mother figure and the pain felt by a child whose parents separated with great animosity.

Symptoms may be activated with disappointment about infertility or ambivalence about your children.

When this tooth is asking for attention
- Look for inner conflict about how you care for and nourish your own body.
- Do you speak to yourself kindly?
- Do you harbor guilty feelings about some behaviour of yours that's affected your health (such as smoking or disordered eating)?
- Consider whether you feel truly worthy of care, kindness or forgiveness.

Daddy archetype:
Upper first premolar (5)

The Daddy tooth represents your desire for attention from an idealized parent who not only provides security and abundance for the family, but who also shows you love, plays with you and backs you to pursue your goals.

The tooth holds energies of compassionate companionship and affectionate confidence in your abilities.

The strength of this tooth lies in feeling worthy: of success, forgiveness, love, patience and attention.

This tooth is vulnerable to feeling held back, either by the absence of a father figure or by the presence of a cold, indifferent father. It can hold onto complicated grief around the loss of a father figure, perhaps embodying an unmet desire to be forgiven, or bearing scars of harsh criticism.

Symptoms may reflect memories (your own or ancestral) of a father who abandoned their children or died young, or of a family where siblings competed ruthlessly for their father's attention.

This tooth can respond to ruminating regretfully about a past relationship if you find yourself swinging again and again between unworthiness and blame.

Symptoms may activate in this tooth if you feel confused about whether you want to be loved or admired, or find yourself trying to earn love and acceptance at the expense of your authenticity.

When this tooth is asking for attention
- Check for where you might be compromising your ideals or safety in unsupportive relationships.
- When you were young was it unsafe to be the favorite child, or was it uncomfortably obvious that you were not the favorite?
- Offer yourself sweet, compassionate forgiveness for your greatest regrets.

- Pay attention to how loveable you are, without needing any outside confirmation.

Friend archetype:
Lower right first premolar (28)

The Friend tooth reflects your relationships with your closest peers, including best friends, close cousins or siblings.

It holds the energy of youthful connections: brothers and sisters you can count on, holidays with cousins, a gang of childhood buddies or a group of college friends.

The strength of this tooth lies in the security of a close-knit group of like-minded peers who allow you to express your individuality.

This tooth is vulnerable to feeling betrayed or being estranged from friends or siblings in relationships that have been lost or distorted over time. It may carry a feeling that you lost a friendship because you weren't good enough, or grief for a shared passion, ability or virtue that you lost along with a departed friend.

Symptoms can reflect nostalgia about a childhood home that was sold or can't be accessed again. The tooth can suffer from missing old friends so much that you can't be happy in your present circumstances.

Tooth 28 can hold memories (your own or ancestral) of a sibling or friend who died when you were both young, or a twin lost before birth. This tooth may remember a sensitive child who couldn't find peace in a large noisy family. It may be activated by the heartbreak of finding out a painful truth about a friend, or be vulnerable to feeling manipulated by a dominant or narcissistic friend.

When this tooth is asking for attention
- Try to reconnect with dear friends you have lost touch with.
- Revisit a place where you used to enjoy fun times with kids the same age as you.

- Do you feel used by your friends?
- Consider how you may need to preserve your privacy and set stronger boundaries within a friendship, even if doing so could risk losing the friendship.

Lover archetype:
Lower left first premolar (21)

The Lover tooth reflects your relationship with a spouse, lover, sweetheart, crush or metamour (polyamorous partner). It may carry desire for unconditional, exclusive, true love.

It holds the energy of your heart, romantic love and erotic passion.

The strength of this tooth lies in experiencing pleasure, satisfaction and happiness; and joyously express how you love yourself and how you look. It thrives when love and lust, heart and hormones, are all in alignment.

This tooth is vulnerable to indifference, hatred, heartbreak, disappointment with dating, soulless casual sex, and loneliness.

Symptoms can be activated by feeling you are only desirable as long as you are useful, attractive or compliant. This tooth suffers from cruel criticism, gaslighting or silent treatment from your lover.

This tooth can hold memories (your own or ancestral) of unrequited or undeclared love, or passionate romance turned loveless marriage.

When this tooth is asking for attention
- Look for where you feel unlovable and rejected especially in the weeks or months before your symptoms appeared.
- Are you secretly still grieving a broken heart from your past?
- Are your needs for respectful love and sexual pleasure being met in your current circumstances?

- Consider what needs to change so you can open your heart to receive love.

Meet your second premolar archetypes

Harvest archetype: Upper left second premolar (13)

The Harvest tooth embodies your understanding that words and actions can have far-reaching, delayed or long-term consequences. It may hold onto your response when the people closest to you don't seem to have your best interests at heart.

It holds the energy of receiving, of karma and repeating cycles of life lessons.

The strength of this tooth lies in living with alignment to your innate talents, natural gifts and intuition. It thrives with taking responsibility for your needs such as when you recognize and respond appropriately to hunger, thirst, tiredness or difficult emotions.

The Harvest tooth is vulnerable to self-sacrifice, self-denial, disassociation and unrealistic expectations of yourself or close relationships. Symptoms may be activated if you blame someone else for your suffering, such as feeling deprived of your partner's time, attention or fidelity.

This tooth can hold memories (your own or ancestral) of couples or families who suffered from separation caused by one member's dishonesty, incompetence or selfishness.

Tooth 13 may be sensitive to collective trauma from being forced to abandon homeland, livelihood or family in order to survive.

When this tooth is asking for attention
- Look for situations where you ignored red flags or let yourself be persuaded against your preferences.
- Do you fear that you will be left by your lover, or feel responsible that a loved one is dying?
- Consider what you might have said or done in the past that you need to take accountability for now.

Alliance archetype:
Upper right second premolar (4)

The Alliance tooth relates to the social dynamics of loss, grief, death, abandonment and betrayal in your life. It holds idealism about friends, colleagues, your children and other relationships.

The energy of this tooth represents the road to hell that was paved with good intentions.

This tooth may be strongest when hopefulness about other people is tempered with well-informed discernment. It can thrive on bringing your creative expression into the public eye.

This tooth is vulnerable to making wishes without taking any action towards manifesting them. It can carry disappointment and despair when your beliefs about other people (including your own children) don't match the reality of their behavior.

Symptoms may be activated by self-punishment for faults you see in yourself or by believing that your ego must be destroyed for spiritual growth.

This tooth can hold memories (your own or ancestral) of a traumatic loss such as widowhood or a divorce you didn't choose. The memory may be of a breakup between parent and child, between business partners or between best friends; any time when you felt that the rupture of your relationship was completely out of your hands.

When this tooth is asking for attention
- Look for relationships in which you are uptight or dogmatic.
- Consider whether feeling ambivalent about your goals is leading to a lack of motivation.
- Have you felt disappointed by reaching a goal that turned out to be the wrong ideal?
- Do you feel as though you are not fulfilling your soul purpose or that a powerful external force is keeping you from your goals?

Trust archetype:
Lower left second premolar (20)

The Trust tooth reflects the kind of relationships that may ground you or limit you. It can hold onto memories of cruel words, silent treatment, or unjust blame from people who are supposed to love you, such as a jealous sibling or spouse.

It represents security, trust and confidence as well as insecurity, resentment, envy and jealousy.

The strength of this tooth is loyalty, tolerance and endurance.

This tooth is vulnerable to situations that keep you stuck in an unhappy status quo without enabling growth, such as distrusting someone you love.

Symptoms may be activated when you are not getting your expectations met, when you give generously to others even though they don't reciprocate, or when you don't follow through on the promises you make to yourself.

This tooth can hold memories (your own or ancestral) of someone who grimly tolerated infidelity or abuse (consciously or unconsciously) or who tried valiantly to hold their family together through an emotionally devastating rupture.

When this tooth is asking for attention
- Look for when you feel betrayed or let down by someone you trusted.
- Try to tune into your body's needs and respond intuitively.
- When you are hungry what do you crave?
- When you are tired during the day do you need a nap or fresh air?
- Do you speak to yourself harshly?

Rival archetype:
Lower left second premolar (29)

The Rival tooth reflects peer relationships, such as siblings, friends, classmates or colleagues at your level. It may carry the memory of an unborn twin or a longing to find your twin flame.

It can hold onto the energy of competition, frustration, resentment, entitlement or bitterness and be scarred by deep depression.

The strength of this tooth is in friendship, camaraderie and companionship with your equals.

This tooth is vulnerable to unfair comparison and competition with a sibling, colleague or friend that left a bad taste in your mouth. Symptoms can be activated by suddenly learning something upsetting about a friend, colleague, sibling, or about yourself.

This tooth can hold memories (your own or ancestral) of having lost a sibling to death, estrangement or lifelong conflicts. It may hold collective memories of suffering from conquest or colonization.

When this tooth is asking for attention
- Look at where you can nurture or repair a peer relationship.
- Try deepening your connections with friends or workmates.
- If you've never had difficulties with these kinds of

relationships, consider whether you feel a part of yourself is holding you back.
- Are you irritated by feeling as though you have a legitimate right to something even though it is inaccessible?

MEET YOUR FIRST MOLAR ARCHETYPES

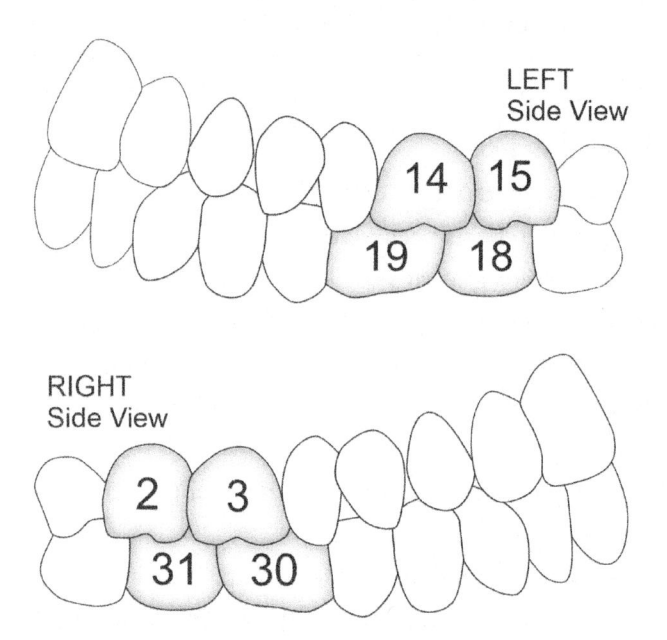

Identifying your molar teeth

Earth Mother archetype: Upper left first molar (14)

The Earth Mother tooth reflects your primary sources for nourishment and support. This tooth reminds you that your body depends on your place in the living systems of the Earth and that your health is inescapably meshed with the health of the planet.

It represents your experience of restoration, relaxation, nourishment and rebalancing.

This tooth holds unconscious beliefs about femininity and

womanhood so how it responds to these themes is affected by your experiences of gender identity and sexuality. It is associated with feeling judged on your appearance or having poor self-image.

The strength of this tooth is in emotional self-expression, balance, empathy and co-operation. It thrives when you feel like you've found the place where you belong on Earth and your needs are easily met.

This tooth is vulnerable to fraught mother-daughter relationships, restrictive diets, negative body image and homelessness. Symptoms may be activated if you choose to eat differently from your friends or you follow an ideological diet despite your cravings. It may carry collective memories of famine.

This tooth can hold memories (your own or ancestral) of a traumatic migration away from homeland and family to a place where what you have to say is ignored, silenced or misinterpreted.

When this tooth is asking for attention
- Look at how well how you meet your own physical, emotional, spiritual and psychological needs.
- Do you have low expectations of having your needs respected by people around you?
- Consider whether you take pride in extreme frugality or restrictive eating.
- Do you make yourself eat food you don't like the taste of so that it isn't wasted?

Sun archetype:
Upper right first molar (3)

The Sun tooth relates to your professional ambitions, and the influence upon your own work life of a father figure's (or ancestor's) occupation, trade or profession. This tooth can embody an inner conflict about work, such as resenting long hours.

This tooth holds unconscious beliefs about masculinity, gender and sexuality so it reacts differently depending on your experiences of gender identity and sexuality.

The strength of this tooth lies in trusting in a higher power in relation to your occupation, such as believing you have a soul purpose, following your intuition to resign, or applying the magic of manifesting to your ambitions.

This tooth is vulnerable to fear (or past experience) of disappointing a father figure or feeling you can never measure up to them. It can hold onto a childhood belief that your father left because you weren't good enough for them.
Symptoms may be activated if you have abandoned a career path that you were passionate about; or lost touch with your deepest convictions and youthful dreams.

This tooth can hold memories (your own or ancestral) of feeling disapproval towards your father's profession or alternatively losing your parents' support because they disapproved of your life choices.

When this tooth is asking for attention
- Look for insights from both sleep dreams and what someone might consider to be unrealistic aspirational dreams.
- Meditate on your life purpose.
- Explore any feelings of being dissatisfied with your chosen career.
- Accept that your beliefs and ideals may be different from what other people in your life expect of you.
- Do you need to reclaim an ambition that is important to your self-image?
- Consider whether you need more sleep.

Professional archetype: Lower right first molar (30)

The Professional tooth relates to your job performance, work environment and relationships with colleagues. It also represents how you first learned about the social expectations you encounter at school or work. It is vulnerable to conflicts between the culture of your school or workplace and the culture of your family.

The strength of this tooth lies in your autonomy, competence, abilities, power and efficiency.

This tooth is vulnerable to imposter syndrome, acting as a spokesperson saying things you don't agree with or being forced to wear a uniform you hate.

This tooth can hold memories (your own or ancestral) of failing to achieve your goals due to lack of financial means, or having your professional ambitions blocked because of gender, race, disability or other factors outside of your control.

It can hold distress arising from the way a father figure or your culture teaches, corrects and criticizes social behaviors. Symptoms may be in response to growing up without praise for, encouragement of, or interest in, your efforts. It may represent a father who was completely absent, or who tried to stop you succeeding.

When this tooth is asking for attention
- Look at what needs to change in your work life.
- This tooth may need you to reconnect with youthful ambitions that you had to abandon for some material reason.
- Consider how you can change your appearance so that it better represents your true self.
- Consider how to follow your bliss and do what brings you pleasure even if it seems professional rewards or recognition would be unattainable.

Home archetype:
Lower left first molar (19)

The Home tooth relates to the romantic partnerships, family and the home that you create for yourself as an adult. It represents the privacy of your personal space and intimate relationships.

It holds the energies of receiving love and support with reciprocity and personal integrity.

The strength of this tooth lies in expressing your authentic identity and desires as an adult. It thrives when you feel welcome as your true self or can be understood in your own language and accent.

This tooth is vulnerable to difficulties with finding or receiving love, struggles with fertility or conflicts around sexual or gender identity. Symptoms may be activated by disrespect, privacy violations, or being forced to say things against your will.

This tooth can hold memories (your own or ancestral) of your home being occupied during a war, or a partner cheating with their lover in your bed, or someone reading your private diary (or cellphone messages) without permission.

When this tooth is asking for attention
- Try changing the way you dress or the design of your home to come more into alignment with your most authentic sense of self.
- Do you feel too proud, or too ashamed, to ask for what you want?
- Does it feel useless to ask for anything because you are not worthy of receiving?
- Try to recognize and name your own deepest emotions and desires.
- Do you need to claim a room of your own?

Meet your second molar archetypes

Night archetype:
Upper left second molar (15)

The Night tooth relates to your mother's family and cultural heritage. It can reflect unresolved grief for death, loss or abandonment.

It holds energies of belonging and exclusion within your extended family.

The strength of this tooth lies in cultural continuity particularly with your maternal heritage, your home, your hometown or your homeland.

This tooth is vulnerable to feeling devalued, abandoned, uninteresting, unworthy or low status.

Symptoms may be activated by a judgmental mother figure, a blood feud, or from feeling like you have chosen the losing side in a conflict.

This tooth can hold memories (your own or ancestral) of being unwanted, marginalized or forgotten by the family especially if you looked different or didn't fit in.

When this tooth is asking for attention
- Look for experiences of loss and grief in the weeks or months leading up to the symptoms starting.
- Try reconnecting with relatives in your mother's family, learning more about the cultural traditions of your maternal lineage, or visiting their homeland.
- Have you been at odds with your family, who made you feel like you were annoying or a misfit?
- Consider whether you deny your own desires and aspirations because they don't fit in with your family's expectations or go against your family's values.

Name archetype:
Upper right second molar (2)

The Name tooth reflects how you measure yourself against the strongest, highest-ranking member of your father's family, your workplace or a social group. It responds to how influential you see yourself within a group or how proud you feel to be part of the group.

This tooth relates to how you identify with your family's name (surname). It may be vulnerable to uncritical reliance on your family lineage rather than your own achievements; or alternatively to a wholesale rejection of your paternal heritage without acknowledging any good qualities. It holds an energy of comparison, status, pride and influence.

The strength of this tooth is in thinking independently and critically.

This tooth is vulnerable to feeling excluded from a valued group to the extent that you will censor your own thoughts if they seem to threaten your sense of belonging. Symptoms can be activated if you feel like your father's family never accepted you.

Beyer associated decay on the biting surface with secrets or uncertainty about who is your real father.

When this tooth is asking for attention

- Look for an unconscious aversion to bearing children who would continue your family lineage.
- Do you criticize yourself for not measuring up to a father figure, or feel uncomfortable about how alike you are?
- Is your personal development inhibited by pride in, or shame for, a social allegiance?
- Consider whether you tend to self-sabotage your efforts to achieve greater professional or social status?

Goals archetype:
Lower right second molar (31)

The Goals tooth relates to your intentions and objectives in relation to anything significant that you are trying to accomplish or conquer. It holds the big picture context for your actions and their results.

It carries the energy of adolescent idealism and professional aspirations when your identity is tied to your achievements. It can reflect pathological perfectionism.

The strength of this tooth lies in your pride, sovereignty and self-confidence. It thrives when you are comfortable with your talents being recognized, your efforts made visible and your successes shared.

This tooth is vulnerable to being the target of racism, sexism, homophobia, or any prejudice that makes you feel held back. Symptoms in this tooth are asking you to stop tolerating those microaggressions that wear you down day after day, and to honor your youthful ideals, hopes and dreams. Symptoms may also be activated if you are unable to get the financial support you need to realize your goals.

This tooth may hold your own, ancestral or collective, resentment about being scapegoated, misjudged, stereotyped, segregated, oppressed or living as a second-class citizen. Alternatively, it can carry the consequences of you, your ancestors or a group you identify with, wielding power unscrupulously.

Beyer associates decay on the cheek-facing surface with wealth that was inherited unexpectedly or sudden fame experienced without effort.

When this tooth is asking for attention
- Look for friction from being misjudged at work, school or in public especially in the weeks or months before you noticed symptoms starting.

- Are you indecisive because you fear the wider impact of your actions?
- Do you feel guilty about sudden wealth or effortless fame?
- Consider whose goals you are pursuing in life now?

Conception archetype: Lower left second molar (18)

The Conception tooth relates to bonds between mother and child, between conscious mind and physical body, and between human and Earth. It may reflect your feelings about your physical appearance.

It can retain the energy of your mother at the time of your conception, their emotions during the pregnancy, and the birth experience. It may carry the long-term consequences of something in the past that led to you feeling rejected.

The strength of this tooth is feeling an unconditional sense of being welcomed and loved, and believing your body is worthy of care.

This tooth is vulnerable to feeling that you are unwanted, your timing is off, or that you are not good enough to belong. Symptoms can be activated if you wish that you hadn't been born or if you have suicidal thoughts.

This tooth can hold memories (your own or ancestral) of a pregnancy considered to be accidental, unplanned, too soon or too late, such as a young, single mother who was punished, publicly shamed or hidden from public view; or a weary mother of a large family who thought she was finished with child-bearing. It may embody experiences of being abandoned, institutionalized, or neglected as a child.

When this tooth is asking for attention
- Look at the circumstances of your conception, gestation and birth.

- Look at your closest relationships and the little annoyances or irritations of everyday life that you tolerate.
- Explore whether you disassociate from experiences of joy and love, or sacrifice your well-being for others.

MEET YOUR WISDOM TEETH ARCHETYPES

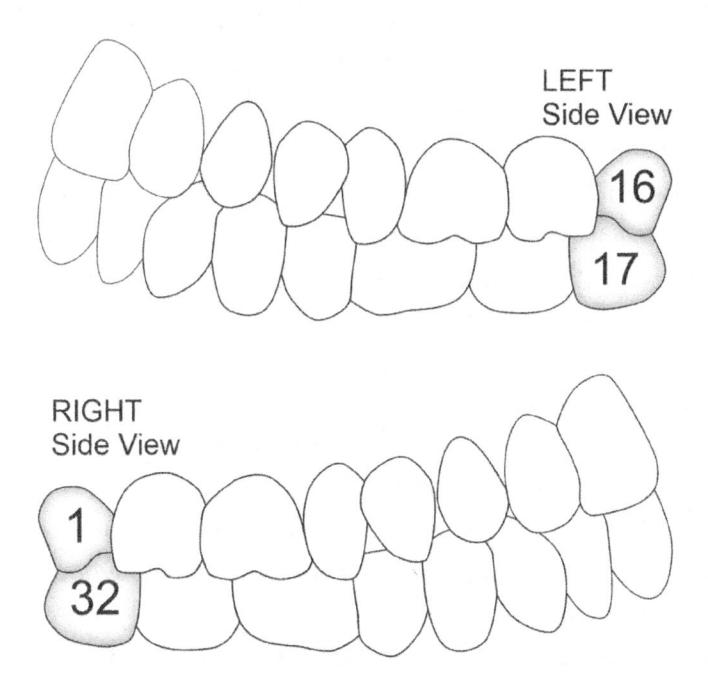

Identifying your wisdom teeth

Virtues archetype:
Upper left wisdom tooth (16)

The Virtues tooth relates to your ancestors' culture, moral code and religious rituals. This tooth reaches far back through your lineage to the original beliefs of your grandmothers (or earlier foremothers) about defining who belongs to the community and who doesn't.

It holds the energy of judging what behaviors and beliefs should be considered right or wrong. It can represent rigid beliefs about hygiene, diet, dress or manners.

The strength of this tooth lies in living with integrity with your own morality. It thrives when you feel safe to speak about your spiritual beliefs and values.

This tooth is vulnerable to suppressing your own thinking to comply with rigid religious obligations, follow an unscrupulous guru or join a cult. Symptoms may be activated by chronic depression, chronic fatigue, or judging your own behavior and language harshly against very strict standards.

This tooth can hold memories (your own or ancestral) of being harmed by your own community's oppressive or exploitative systems that denied your humanity. It may carry memories of conflict with the teachings of religious leaders, or of feeling stressed or isolated for atheist beliefs.

When this tooth is asking for attention
- Consider when you feel guilt or shame for your own behavior or other people's.
- Do you live in fear of being criticized, punished, or cancelled for activities that could be considered excessive, self-harming or debauched?
- Do you find yourself silently judging other people's personal habits even if they don't affect you directly?

Lore archetype:
Upper right wisdom tooth (1)

The Lore tooth relates to your ancestors' laws and religious teachings. This tooth reaches far back into the archaic times represented in the earliest stories and legends of your grandfather's culture.

This tooth holds systems and structures for making sense of the world such as laws, rules, expectations, etiquette or social norms, including gender expression. It can reflect your feelings about religious protocols or leaders.

The strength of this tooth lies in an existential search for the nature of your soul and awareness of the natural or spiritual world. It thrives when you are sincere and honest about your soul's path and authentic identity.

This tooth is vulnerable to unexamined privilege and cultural appropriation; or alternatively, to feeling like you don't measure up to your family's status or identity.

Symptoms may be activated if you are in conflict with relatives who are proudly preserving their social status by controlling other family members' behavior, thinking, political affiliations or occupation.

This tooth can carry collective memories of domination or exploitation, especially in your paternal lineage. It may be asking you to recognize and honor what's been lost from your cultural heritage and distant ancestors.

It can be vulnerable to feeling ambivalent about studying other spiritual traditions or changing your religious affiliation (e.g. converting to marry or advance professionally).

When this tooth needs attention
- Look for when you may have abandoned a soul-aligned practice because it seemed like a waste of time.
- Consider your relationship with oppressive belief systems such as colonialism, classism, sexism, racism, homophobia, ableism, ageism etc.
- Do you feel like a spiritual hypocrite?
- Do you fear you've lost touch with your soul?

Mystic archetype:
Lower right wisdom tooth (32)

The Mystic tooth relates to the material aspects of your spiritual path or journey of self-discovery, including physiological practices such as mindful breathing, meditation, plant medicine, entering trance states and so on.

It holds energies of introspection and authenticity.

The strength of this tooth lies in learning and practicing disciplines that shape a natural, simple spiritual life. These may require living in alignment with values such as generosity, kindness and honesty.

This tooth thrives when you speak truthfully from your heart, wholeheartedly share what you have and forgive yourself unconditionally.

This tooth is vulnerable to sacrificing your physical well-being for spiritual ideals e.g. excessive fasting or tithing.

Symptoms can be activated by pretentious compliance with spiritual practices, social conventions or by performing a role at odds with your real beliefs and values.

This tooth can hold memories (your own or ancestral) of a young person who was physically or socially harmed by their passionate commitment to extreme religious or spiritual practices.

When this tooth is asking for attention
- Look for when you feel like you are keeping a stiff upper lip, living a lie or keeping a painful secret.
- Try meditation, philanthropy or volunteering at a local homeless shelter.
- Consider whether your spiritual practices involve cultural appropriation, gaslighting or hypocrisy.
- Do you use good manners or compulsive behaviors to hide unhappiness?

Honor archetype:
Lower left wisdom tooth (17)

The Honor tooth relates to your maternal grandmother and her foremothers' traditions for protecting the lineage of mitochondrial DNA connecting mother to daughter, from the first human mother all the way through to you. It can carry the energy of a mother in your lineage who tried to force her children into a life path they didn't want.

The strength of this tooth lies in self-reflective, self-aware thinking. It thrives when you listen to your intuition and soul's calling.

This tooth is vulnerable to secrecy, lying or shame or inner conflict about moral beliefs that limit your freedom.

This tooth can hold memories (your own or ancestral) of unplanned, unwanted pregnancy, abortion or adoption, and believing your family was ashamed of you. It may carry the residue of being judged immoral by the customs of an ancestor's time and place; or embarrassment about your mother's behaviours or housekeeping.

When this tooth is asking for attention
- Consider when you fear rejection or if you are a victim of bullying, oppression or gaslighting.
- Do you feel conscious or unconscious shame about your sexuality, customs, food, hygiene or household habits?
- Are you, or someone close to you, so nostalgic for the good old days that it stops you living fully in the present moment?

10.

SYMPTOMS AS MESSENGERS

This chapter includes a directory of metaphysical interpretations for common categories of symptoms that can occur in the mouth. Some oral health symptoms may come to your attention with uncomfortable sensations or visual cues such as color changes or swelling. In other cases you may remain blithely unaware that anything is amiss until a dentist's specialist equipment and training identifies a serious problem below the surface.

However, nearly all oral health problems start almost imperceptibly, with the equivalent of a whisper or a gentle nudge that may be easily ignored. If you pay attention to your mouth and respond quickly to an occasional twinge of sensitivity to ice water, or a rare spot of blood when you floss, then you are more likely to be able to relieve those symptoms quickly and completely. But amongst the clamor and demands of daily life, it's easy to disregard subtle signs until your body turns up the dial.

When sensitivity turns into toothache or bleeding gums develop into gingivitis, it may still be realistic to effectively stop symptoms from escalating. At that point resolution may take longer to achieve and dental interventions may be harder to avoid, but it could be possible.

Unfortunately, the longer you try to ignore your symptoms, the more likely they are to become increasingly aggressive. Don't wait for unbearable pain, unsightly damage or an extensive, expensive treatment plan to start taking effective action.

Right now is always the best time to pay attention to what the symptoms in your teeth and gum are trying to tell you. No matter how serious or trivial your oral health issues are, you'll get a better outcome if you try to understand the root cause and what response your body needs. Try to approach problems with relaxed curiosity about their origins rather than anxiety about the future.

Discussions about disease that attribute ill health to individual choices or actions are problematic because they often disregard the importance of factors which are out of the individual's control. For example, the possible physical factors influencing your oral health could include genetics, the oral microbiome that you acquired at birth, global and local food systems, environmental toxins, physical trauma, the impacts of technology on oral posture and many more.

Blaming individuals for their ill health also disregards the metaphysical relevance of family culture, collective trauma, social prejudices, unjust economics and more. I believe that illness is intersectional, meaning one or more physical factors can interact with one or more metaphysical factors. I believe that metaphysical influences rarely lead to ill health unless there are also physical factors, and visa versa. That's why not everyone who eats sugar gets tooth decay, and not everyone who grew up with childhood trauma has cavities.

Because oral health symptoms rarely have a single cause you are likely to get better oral health outcomes by exploring and responding to metaphysical influences along with physical remedies, protocols or interventions. However, relying only on metaphysical strategies for healing can be risky, and even life threatening in some circumstances. How can you tell when it's appropriate to invest more in physical or metaphysical healing?

WEIGHTING METAPHYSICAL VS. PHYSICAL INFLUENCES

There is no one-size-fits-all system to tease out a symptom's (comparatively) straightforward physical cause-and-effect from the more indirect influence of metaphysical factors. Different people may have quite different combinations of interrelated influences for identical symptoms. Furthermore, the relative influence of metaphysical and physical factors may alter over your lifetime and with changing circumstances.

With discernment on a case-by-case basis, you may be able to make an approximate guess at how much attention to give metaphysical causes and how much time, effort and resources should be directed towards physical remedies.

Metaphysical interpretations may be most helpful when you don't have a clear diagnosis or when a second opinion is contradictory. They are least risky when your symptoms are minor or fleeting. With symptoms that are both minor and ambiguous, the benefits of prioritizing metaphysical understanding over physical interventions are more likely to outweigh the risks.

When your symptoms are serious or do have an obvious physical explanation, conventional dental treatment and/or home remedies and lifestyle changes are probably necessary. In such cases a metaphysical approach should be considered complementary rather than wholly sufficient. Dental interventions can be more reliably effective, fast acting and uncomplicated when you also work with the underlying energetic answers to 'why you', 'why now', and 'why in this part of your mouth'.

The symptoms in your teeth and gums draw attention to any areas in your life that aren't in alignment with your highest good or life purpose. You are a beautiful, bright shining manifestation of the Universe (or God, Life, or Love). The human condition means we don't always feel or act like that though. Nature and nurture, ancestry and environment, free will and systemic oppression all conspire to divert us from embodying our essential truth consistently.

A holistic approach to oral health symptoms that addresses the metaphysical influences is likely to heal more than just your teeth and gums. The motivation to improve your teeth or gum health can help break through blocks to changing unhelpful behavioral patterns or releasing suppressed or distorted emotions, with the happy side effect of improving your general well-being.

DIRECTORY OF ORAL HEALTH ISSUES

Abscesses and infections

A dental abscess starts as a localized infection inside a tooth, an area of gum, or jawbone, which provokes an inflammatory immune response from your body. Eventually a pocket of pus (cyst) may start to erode the healthy tissue around it, which is when infection becomes an abscess. Abscesses may develop very slowly over a long period or burst into your awareness suddenly and painfully. At that point they are a serious symptom requiring a swift intervention.

Abscesses may show up as shiny, red, swollen gums or redness and swelling in your face. They can feel like an intense throbbing pain that may spread to your ear, jaw or neck and feel worse when you lie down, or from hot or cold food and drinks. They may cause a bad taste in your mouth or bad breath.

If your abscess develops into a fever, a loose tooth or difficulty opening your mouth, swallowing, or breathing, you should seek dental or medical attention immediately. Don't take a wait-and-see approach!

Left untreated, an abscess can erode your jawbone, gum tissue or tooth root, leading to tooth loss, gum recession or jawbone cavitation. In some cases, the infection can escape its local cyst and travel through the lymph or blood to infect or inflame other organs, which may lead to autoimmune conditions and in some cases death.

Interpreting an abscess or infection: Are you angry?
An abscess may represent suppressed feelings of anger, rage, resentment or frustration.

Chronic abscesses could be the embodiment of a pattern of love-hate relationships, ruminating on injustices, or having internal conversations in which you repeatedly try to defend yourself to an imaginary listener.

If an unusual abscess has just appeared, then a conflict may be coming to a head with someone.

Try somatic techniques (see Chapter 11) to help you get out of your head and be more connected with your body. If you are in a toxic relationship or workplace, the abscess may be asking you to leave, or at least get help to improve your current circumstances.

For a more nuanced understanding, check the associations for the nearest teeth and meridians, and explore whether you feel angry or frustrated in relation to those themes.

See also *root problems* and *gum conditions*.

Ankylosed tooth (immobile tooth)
A tooth is ankylosed when the root is permanently connected to the jawbone due to a lack of periodontal ligament. To the naked eye, an ankylosed tooth doesn't generally appear unusual although sometimes it may be a little shorter or taller than the rest of your teeth. It's most likely to be diagnosed if you get braces

because an ankylosed tooth cannot move. Dentists aren't sure what can cause the periodontal ligament to dissolve, but most believe that physical trauma (including a crooked bite) may be involved.

Interpreting an ankylosed tooth: Are you inflexible?
An ankylosed tooth may represent suppressed fear, manifesting as a need to feel in control. This symptom may be drawing your attention to compulsive repetitive behaviors.

Try nervous system regulation techniques (see Chapter 11 for suggestions) to help you feel safe enough to be more flexible in your thinking and responses.

For a more nuanced understanding, look for instances of fearful rigid thinking in relation to that tooth's archetype.

See also *gum problems (periodontal ligament)*.

Bruxism, jaw clenching and TMJD (temporomandibular joint disorder)

The lower jaw is connected to the upper jawbone by the TMJ (temporomandibular joint). The TMJ is a powerful, flexible, complex mechanism which appears deceptively simple, but it can hold a lot of tension.

Bruxism refers to grinding or clenching your jaws. Stress is a common factor for bruxism, especially in adults. However, genetics, oral posture, mouth breathing, internal parasites, allergies, heavy metal toxicity, some medications and some medical conditions may also trigger bruxism. It's important to identify and address any possible physical factors, as well as working on stress or other metaphysical influences.

Bruxism usually occurs while asleep, so many people remain unaware that they are clenching or grinding until someone else points it out, often a dentist observing effects on your teeth such as wear and tear, cracks or chips. Severe bruxism can actually cause the teeth foundations to be loosened and the teeth to fall out. Other consequences of bruxism include sore jaw muscles, earaches or headaches near the jaw joint, problems opening and closing the jaw, or heightened tooth sensitivity.

Dentists commonly prescribe an appliance such as a mouthguard or night guard to help protect the teeth from the effects of grinding. While mouthguards can help prevent enamel from cracking, chipping and wear, they don't deal with the cause of the tension and sometimes wearing a mouthguard can actually cause additional discomfort or damage.

Interpreting bruxism: Do you feel powerless?
Dharni had started grinding her teeth for the first time early in 2020 while recovering from stressful knee surgery. It wasn't long before the bruxism caused one of her molars (tooth 29, the Professional archetype) to crack around an old filling. Even after being refilled the tooth continued to be hypersensitive.

The TMJ joint, connecting upper and lower jaws, represents the connection between desires and actions. As such it can embody fears, impulsiveness or hesitation about acting on your intentions. Symptoms such as TMJ disorder, a clicking jaw or teeth grinding (bruxism) may indicate unconscious irritation or frustration related to current or past circumstances. Bruxism may be caused by the stress of feeling powerless, bullied or intimidated.

Dharni had worked hard to build a career out of her passion for social and environmental sustainability. Working as an advocate inside a multinational corporation, she was often arguing a minority position against short-term business priorities. The corporate culture ground onwards, grinding her spirit down. She lacked the support to be able to express herself authentically and help create real change.

Dharni dreamed of redirecting her career into the meaningful regeneration of land and communities. But she wasn't sure how to find the right opportunity and relied on the security and income from her current job. Although there were plenty of personal and collective stressors accumulating in 2020, Dharni noticed that her bruxism and TMJ pain would reduce whenever she could take time off from her demanding career.

Like many people, she found that working from home during Covid-19 lockdowns made it too easy to spend every waking moment on the job. One of the most difficult aspects of this for her was having no respite from speaking up in video meetings and presentations despite her constantly painful jaw.

A new bruxism habit may be embodying how you're coping with feeling stuck in a disempowering workplace or relationship. However, when grinding has been a lifelong habit, your jaws may be asking for you to address childhood anger that wasn't acceptable or safe for you to express at the time.

After facing another health challenge (an ankle injury) during the same couple of difficult years with her jaw, Dharni decided it was time to listen more deeply to her body. In 2022, she asked her employer for a six-month sabbatical which she used to focus on healing and learning. Her jaw pain reduced significantly, and she confidently returned to eating hard foods (something she had given up because of the jaw pain). She still wears a mouthguard a few days a week to protect her teeth, and is currently exploring different possibilities for developing a new career that builds on her gifts and passions.

See also *cracked, chipped and broken teeth*.

Canker sores (aphthous ulcers)

Canker sores are shallow, small lesions that appear on the inside of your cheeks or lips, or on your tongue. They are not usually serious or long lasting but they can be very uncomfortable.

Canker sores are not to be confused with cold sores caused by the herpes virus which tend to occur on the outside of your lips.

Canker sores may be caused by a minor injury to the soft tissue inside your mouth, or by diet, stress, immune or inflammation conditions, menstrual hormones, or using a toothpaste or mouthwash containing sodium lauryl sulfate (SLS). They are more common in young people and women.

Interpreting canker sores: What do you need to say?

Canker sores can be a sign that you are trying to cover up feeling overwhelmed, exhausted or stressed out. If you get canker sores frequently then you may have a pattern of helping other people at the expense of your health, personal priorities, or inner resources.

Canker sores may appear when you are presenting a friendly, helpful image but inside you feel like a seething swamp of bitter resentment. They can hold an energy of censoring yourself and biting your tongue rather than saying what you are really thinking. Canker sores may show up when you have taken the blame for someone else's shortcomings without defending yourself (Rose).

Cracking, chipping or breaking teeth

When teeth start cracking, chipping or breaking it's usually from one or more of the following common physical causes:
- a physical trauma (accident, attack or dental intervention) has impacted the integrity of the tooth structure.
- demineralization (caused by stress, undernourishment or high blood sugar).
- bruxism (clenching and grinding).

Depending on where they appear in the mouth, chipped, cracked or broken teeth can impair your ability to chew, speak clearly or smile confidently. They may also cause increased sensitivity, or even severe toothache if the nerve is exposed.

Small chips may do little more than irritate the tongue or inner cheek, but larger chips, cracks and breaks can allow infection inside the tooth, gum or jawbone. If left untreated such infections may lead to autoimmune conditions or other serious, systemic diseases.

Interpreting cracking, chipping or breaking teeth: Are you feeling overwhelmed?
The metaphysical meaning of a chipped, cracked or broken tooth can often be understood by looking broadly at the circumstances of your life during the time in which the damage took place.

Sometimes the connection can be as obvious as a tooth chipping during an argument with someone representing that tooth's archetype. More often the damage happens during or shortly after a stressful period when themes of the tooth's archetype or adjacent meridian were stirred up.

Explore connections between your emotional state that day and any relationships or social situations making you uncomfortable that week. Zoom out further to consider whether you were grappling with any major life decisions that month or feeling worn down by grief or stress that year.

See also *decay (caries and cavities)*, *sensitive teeth* and *root problems*.

Decay (caries and cavities)

Tooth decay is a complex and progressive disease. Caries occurs when areas of tooth enamel (the hard outside layer of a tooth) or dentin (a softer layer underneath the enamel) become compromised and vulnerable to bacteria, which actively break down the tooth structure even further.

When decay appears on the surface of tooth enamel, it shows as a darker color than healthy enamel and can feel comparatively soft when prodded. Decay below the surface is often much larger than what is visible on the surface and is only observable with a dental x-ray or when the tooth is drilled open.

Cavities are holes in enamel that may begin with decay, demineralization, chips or cracks. Many people get shallow cavities in the enamel only (never reaching the dentin) which naturally appear and disappear without any intervention. Deeper cavities into the dentin layer can make the nerve in the center of the tooth feel more sensitive or painful. Both shallow and deep cavities can trap food particles, which feed the decay-causing bacteria.

Interpreting decay and cavities: What is unresolved?

Cavities represent a loss, an absence or the breakdown of boundaries. A tooth may respond with caries when there is conflict or deficiency resulting from interactions with a person who embodies the tooth's archetype.

When you experience tooth decay, your system is pointing out where the adaptive strategies you learned as a child (in order to cope with difficult situations and relationships) are no longer supporting your highest good. These strategies are expressed through your personality and habits, which makes them difficult to observe and change.

Just as a small cavity in the enamel can conceal a much larger area of decay in the dentin, a minor personality quirk may represent a quagmire of unresolved trauma. Decay developing beneath an existing filling can embody denied, or ignored, emotional issues. When you are trying to remineralize tooth decay it can be helpful to try to become more conscious of long-standing adaptive emotional patterns that are no longer serving your well-being.

See also *root problems, sensitive teeth,* and *tooth surfaces.*

Gum conditions (gingivitis, periodontitis, receding gums, gum pockets and bone loss)

Gum symptoms may be caused by a viral or bacterial infection, an autoimmune response, bruxism, stress, dry mouth, excess tartar or even rough toothbrushing. There is no clear definition of gum disease so I don't work with specific metaphysical interpretations for periodontal diagnosis (e.g. gingivitis or periodontitis).

Instead, I refer to the metaphysical themes associated with whichever of the four main types of periodontal tissue are symptomatic: the gingiva, cementum, periodontal ligament or alveolar bone (See Chapter 2 for more detailed physical descriptions of each tissue type).

Mild gum conditions may not cause discomfort but if left untreated they can lead to the uncontrolled infection and inflammation diagnosed as periodontal disease, which increase the risk of suffering from a wide range of other health issues, including pneumonia, heart disease, autoimmune diseases, cancer, and more.

Gingiva (the surface layer of gum tissue) may become red and swollen with gingivitis, a mild, or early stage, of periodontal disease. However, gum disease often begins with gum recession or gum pockets, which cause damage to the tissues below the gingiva, compromising the cementum and periodontal ligaments, which connect the tooth roots to the jawbone.

You may notice your gums receding when the gum tissues shrink to expose the roots of your teeth and show gaps between teeth. Gum recession can happen with, or without, the development of gum pockets, which occur when the gum pulls away from the tooth root to create a gap, or pocket, which can become a food trap, and a home for unhelpful bacteria.

Bone loss is a reduction of the density or thickness of the alveolar bone, which is an extension of the jawbone where it narrows to form sockets that hold teeth roots in place. Bone loss undermines the foundations that support softer gum tissues, causing recession. Severe bone loss can loosen teeth enough for them to fall out.

Interpreting gum problems: Do you lack support?
Lisa came to me with severely receding gums, deep pockets and sensitivity in her upper left gums (around teeth 13, 14 and 15). She had been following her dentist's recommendation to have her gums deep cleaned four times a year. When this schedule was interrupted by Covid lockdowns, Lisa started coaching with me for a more optimized home care approach.

She told me that at her last dental cleaning 'the dentists said my gum pocket depth has reduced, which is good. But still, I always feel like nothing I do is ever enough. It always seems as though he's unfairly disappointed in me. Like he doesn't believe that I floss and brush just the way he recommends.'

Gum issues may represent confusion between who you are (your conscious identity) and what you are (your unconscious body). This inner conflict can lead to indecision, poor social or energetic boundaries or a lack of self-belief, making you feel frustration, resentment, fear or regret. When you suppress or deny these feelings, your emotions can become embodied into gum symptoms.

When I asked Lisa to focus on her physical sensations as she remembered the dentist's criticism there was a pulsing on the left side of her body (where all her dental problems concentrate): her shoulder was tight, her head and teeth ached.

'Oh, my teeth feel sad,' she exclaimed. She told me that the sadness reminded her of how she felt when thinking about her family's early responses to her body. 'When I was born my father, who was expecting a boy, misheard the doctor and felt excited until it turned to crushing disappointment when he realized I was a girl. Also, my half-Mexican mother was not welcomed by my white paternal grandmother who was very worried that I would be born dark-skinned.'

Lisa was shamed and criticized throughout her childhood for being clumsy or careless, when in fact her behaviour was age-appropriate, but her babysitters had been neglectful. For example, she had been blamed for crawling into a pool and almost drowning at six months and for running, slipping and smashing her face into a wall at four years old.

Mild gum symptoms may be influenced by something that you said (or didn't say) that affected the outcome of a stressful situation. They can flare up when you fear receiving harsh criticism, upsetting your family or being rejected.

Severe gum symptoms may escalate when you (or your ancestors) didn't just fear, but felt, attack from loved ones or community. Severe symptoms can be the embodiment of feeling undermined, devalued and disempowered.

Sexuality and gingiva

Gingiva, the visible pink wet surface of the gum is almost as sensitive as the skin covering your genitals and is also infused with sexual and creative energy. Gingivitis may be an embodiment of inappropriate, inadequate or unbalanced sexual expression. Receding gingiva may be calling you to overcome anything getting in the way of proudly and openly owning your sexuality.

The health of your gingiva can also more broadly represent how authentically the image you present to the world is aligned with your inner truth.

Truth and cementum
Cementum may embody any feelings that you don't acknowledge to yourself, let alone talk about or act upon more publicly. It can represent the security of your energetic boundaries, embodying how consistently you protect yourself from unreasonable expectations or narcissistic demands. Gum pockets opening up as cementum breaks down around certain teeth may reflect conscious or unconscious dishonesty in relation to those tooth archetypes.

Grace and periodontal ligament
The periodontal ligament is associated with your ability to adapt to changing circumstances with grace. Periodontal ligaments provide an energetic buffer against the pressure of the outside world. They can represent your capacity to communicate effectively and use appropriate language for the context. Thinning gums could indicate that you have been unable to advocate effectively for your own interests, or that you don't feel worthy of support.

Support and bone loss
The alveolar part of the jawbone represents your inner strength and alignment with your soul purpose or values. Bone loss may be the embodiment of feeling that you aren't well supported in your life. When periodontitis has eroded the alveolar bone, your social or economic foundation feels insecure or perhaps you feel like you can't trust anyone to have your best interests at heart.

With acute bone loss your gums may be responding to a current or recent situation in which you have felt unsupported, such as a job loss, a break-up or social isolation.

Early onset or chronic bone loss may indicate that you didn't feel well supported by your parents or caregivers when you were growing up. Or perhaps you have a sense that the community or society that you live in doesn't support your existence, because of economic injustice or systemic racism or sexism, homophobia or transphobia. Bone loss can embody an existential sense that the Universe or God isn't really supporting you.

See also *abscesses and infections, ankylosed tooth, bruxism, canker sores, missing teeth, plaque and tartar,* and *sensitive teeth.*

Missing teeth

Adults can have one or more permanent teeth missing for various reasons. Many people never develop the germs for all thirty-two adult teeth, meaning the adult tooth can never grow (hypodontia). Sometimes teeth loosen and fall out spontaneously as a consequence of severe malnutrition, gum disease or bone loss. Teeth can also be lost to a physical trauma such as an accident, deliberate violence or dental misadventure.

Dentists usually only choose to extract unhealthy teeth as a last resort, either because they cannot be saved with other dental interventions or because it's a less expensive treatment than root canals or crowns. Wisdom teeth are the exception as they are commonly extracted to prevent or treat impaction, infection or cavities, because dentists often see wisdom teeth as expendable, in addition to being awkward to clean, drill and fill.

Orthodontists may extract healthy teeth (typically premolars in teenagers) to make more room for crooked teeth to be straightened by braces.

Tooth loss as an adult can distort your speech and compromise your ability to chew food. The jawbone may erode where a tooth was extracted, changing the shape of your face. These problems can be mitigated with an implant (a permanent false tooth embedded in the jawbone), or dentures; usually a fixed bridge attached to remaining stable teeth or a partial bridge, which is a removable false tooth (or row of teeth) supported by other teeth. When all the teeth are missing from one or both jaws, they may be replaced by removable dentures, or a combination of implants and dentures.

Interpreting missing teeth: What is absent?
Socially isolated people have an average of 2.1 fewer natural teeth and lose their teeth 1.4 times more than those with more social contact (Qi et al). However, the energetic impact of a missing tooth is very different if extracted as opposed to never having grown in.

If the tooth germ never developed and the tooth never had a chance to grow, then the archetype of the missing tooth may help you identify an ancestral trauma or family pattern of absence. Alternatively, that part of your mouth may embody the residual energy of your mother's health, emotional state and circumstances while pregnant with you.

If a chronic oral health problem leads to tooth loss later in your life, then there may still be a residue of blocked or unbalanced energy present in the local gum, jaw (or some other part of your body), unless you intentionally addressed the energetic influences at the time of the extraction. Energy issues lingering after an extraction can influence problems with the adjacent teeth, or with an implant on that site, or could contribute to a cavitation developing inside the jawbone.

Dreams about losing teeth are common and Carl Jung interpreted them as the dreamer's fear of losing grip on reality, relationships or self-control (especially during pregnancy). Missing teeth dreams can also symbolize your feelings about growing older.

See also *gum problems, ankylosed teeth, retained baby teeth, mouth meridians, tooth archetypes* and *tooth types* of the missing teeth.

Retained baby teeth

Most people's baby teeth (aka milk or deciduous teeth) start to loosen, and then fall out naturally, from the age of five. They are displaced by adult teeth (aka permanent teeth) growing up deeper inside the jaw then pushing the baby teeth out.

Sometimes, one or more adult teeth never grow in the jawbone, and so sometimes the baby tooth is able to remain stable (albeit small) in a line-up of adult teeth. Other times the adult tooth is present but doesn't grow straight enough to displace the baby tooth. These adult teeth can appear in the gum above or below, in front or behind the retained baby teeth.

Interpreting retained baby teeth: What's unappealing about growing up?

Baby teeth that don't fall out on schedule may represent attachment to either the dependencies, or the freedoms, of childhood. If adulthood looks like hard work (or a scary, dangerous place) then retained baby teeth may embody a reluctance or resistance to growing up and taking on adult risks and responsibilities.

Baby teeth may also be delayed if you have a dominant parent who wants you to stay under their control or a beloved parent whose well-being seems to be tied to your immaturity.

If an adult tooth never grew inside your gum, identify the missing tooth's archetype and consider how that energy is present (or absent) in your family history. You can also identify the nearest meridians to the retained baby tooth and work with those energies.

See also *missing teeth, mouth meridians* and the *tooth archetypes* and *tooth types* of a missing adult tooth.

Root problems (nerve damage, non-vital tooth or resorption)

Root problems are often excruciatingly painful, yet sometimes may be quite painless when the nerve is compromised suddenly. Root pain is not always localized, because the nerves can feel aggravated across a much larger area than the root of the threatened tooth.

You may not recognize this discomfort as a toothache at first. You may experience a headache, throbbing temples, sinus pain, a sore jaw, or earache for the first few days or hours. Unfortunately, the diffuseness of such pain doesn't make it any more bearable, just more difficult to pinpoint the cause.

If the pain persists, it usually eventually becomes more localized. If you put up with intense root pain for long enough it might even stop hurting. Unfortunately, this may mean the nerve has died rather than being spontaneously healed. Also called a 'non-vital tooth' this diagnosis means the pulp, which is made up of blood vessels, nerves and other tissues is either injured or infected to the point where there is no blood flow into the tooth anymore.

Roots can become damaged from the crown down, as when a cavity or crack (or a dentist's drill accidentally) extends through the enamel and dentin to touch the pulp at the center of the tooth, connecting directly into the nerve. Roots can die from the bottom up, as when an infection develops inside the gum, near the base of a tooth root, or when resorption caused by demineralization shrinks the root towards the tooth's crown. Roots can also fail from the inside as a result of physical trauma such as bruxism or being knocked out of alignment.

Root problems sometimes show up on an x-ray as a dark area of infection inside the gum or jaw around the root, or as a shortened root. Dentists will tap on the tooth or use a cold test to see how much sensation the nerve is still picking up to determine whether the tooth can be saved.

Interpreting root problems: How are you displaced?
Roots of teeth play an energetic role in grounding you. They are particularly vulnerable to experiences that disconnect you from your ancestors, family or homeland. When you feel uprooted geographically, it is as though your roots try to help you stay grounded by shouldering more of the energetic responsibility for connecting you to the Earth.

Your roots can be affected by any circumstance in which you feel like you don't belong where you are. When there are difficult emotions and prolonged stress associated with travel or moving house, those circumstances can aggravate old traumas, or old patterns of separation anxiety first experienced in your infancy and stored in the energetic storehouses of your teeth.

Fast travel that disconnects you from the surface of the earth and moves you across time zones in hours instead of days, is potentially particularly hard on teeth roots. Moving house, even within the same town, can stress them too. Periods of homelessness, whether actually living on the streets or couch surfing, can be made more uncomfortable by toothache when you are least resourced to resolve it.

However, you don't have to be geographically displaced for your tooth roots to be vulnerable. Collective experiences of urbanization and migration have eroded whole cultures' relationships with the Earth. This may affect you most if you don't have any historical family ties to the place you live, or lack awareness of its indigenous history. Living in a high-rise apartment block can be hard on the teeth of some sensitive people. Roots can also respond to being surrounded by people who don't understand or respect you, and they can embody a lack of belief in yourself and hope your future.

You can help to support your roots by sinking into a deeper energetic connection with the land where you live right now. Try leaving the building, getting off the pavement and out of your shoes to connect your body with the Earth. Try eating more locally grown food or even better, getting your hands into the soil to grow your own food. If you are not indigenous to the place you live, learn what you can about how to respect the original culture.

See also *abscesses, decay and cavities, missing teeth* and *tooth archetypes*.

Plaque and tartar

Plaque develops when some of the microorganisms that live in your mouth start to get too comfortable on the surface of your tooth enamel, forming a film. Most plaque-causing bacteria are harmless when they're a minority among the free-floating elements of your oral microbiome. But when they have the opportunity to settle down where yummy food residues (i.e. sugars and carbohydrates) get stuck, they start setting up campgrounds. In cozy nooks and crannies they reproduce themselves to create an expansive sticky surface designed to catch more unswallowed bits of food. If left to their own devices, communities of well-nourished plaque bacteria may eventually calcify into solid cities of tartar along your gumline and between your teeth.

Different hues and textures of tartar are produced by different kinds of bacteria. Tartar provides a textured surface for more bacteria to stick to, along with more food residues. Bacteria that can cause decay (or gum disease) usually find it hard to get established on the slippery surface of healthy tooth enamel in a constant state of remineralization; but they find a warm welcome on tartar.

Plaque is only really a problem insofar as it's a precursor to tartar, and tartar is problematic because it can contribute to the development of gum recession and gum pockets, as well as providing a welcoming environment for other, even more damaging and aggressive bacteria that cause decay and cavities.

Some tartar is clingier than others, but it's all pretty difficult to remove, and so there is a specialized profession of dental hygienists devoted to this task.

Interpreting plaque and tartar: Are you stuck?
Metaphysically, plaque may represent an over reliance on old habits that are past their use by date. Ask yourself where you are clinging to social or emotional structures such as relationships, work or beliefs that allow, or contribute to, an imbalance in your life.

Plaque and tartar can appear in your mouth when you are overwhelmed or hyper-vigilant. These bacterial communities on your teeth may embody feelings of guilt, regret or self-punishment. If severe tartar runs in your family, or appears on a child's teeth, consider whether these themes were present for your parents, grandparents, or more distant ancestors.

See also *tooth archetypes* and *tooth surfaces* to interpret the specific locations of tartar.

Sensitive teeth
Teeth can feel sensitive to hot or cold temperatures, sweetness, acidity or pressure.

Sensitive teeth may show up as a mild discomfort or stop you in your tracks when you eat, drink, brush, floss or even when you breathe cold air through your mouth. Tooth sensitivity can feel like a sharp electric shock or a thud of dull pain but it usually passes within a few minutes.

Sensitivity can be caused by the presence of an exposed cavity, crack or decay, gum recession, gum pockets or gum disease. Sensitivity is sometimes the harbinger of root problems brewing, or a side effect of demineralization, decay or receding gums.

The most common remedy for sensitivity is toothpaste for

sensitive teeth, which traditionally contained an analgesic to numb the nerve but which does little to remineralize tooth enamel, reverse cavities or regenerate gum tissue, thus potentially masking the message without addressing the cause.

Interpreting sensitive teeth: Are you sensitive?
Tooth sensitivity may be a first whisper, trying to draw your attention to where you are not living in alignment with your highest good. Sensitive teeth embody where you seem to be more vulnerable than other people with similar experiences or circumstances.

If a specific tooth is sensitive, look at its archetype, and nearby meridians. Your tooth may be pointing to relationships or situations in which you need to understand more about your own vulnerability or alternatively, where you lack the necessary sensitivity to interpret nuanced communication.

If your whole mouth is sensitive, it may indicate that you are so overwhelmed by stress that you have shut down emotionally and only your teeth can feel anything anymore.

See also *cracking, chipping or breaking teeth, decay, gum conditions, root problems* and *tooth surfaces*.

Part III: A Toolkit

Any sufficiently advanced technology is indistinguishable from magic.
Arthur C. Clarke's Third Law

11.

TREASURY OF TRANSFORMATIVE TOOLS

The underlying emotional, energetic or psychological influences on your symptoms can point the way to more effective lifelong healing, maintenance and prevention. Yet, in order to respond to the real needs of your teeth and gums, it is not sufficient to just read interpretations. Now it's time for you to lift your eyes from the map and prepare to step into the territory of your own life and body.

This chapter introduces a selection of the most effective and accessible metaphysical practices, exercises and resources that have helped my clients to address their oral health issues. However, almost any modality for emotional or energetic healing can be used in conjunction with the concepts in this book, so feel free to apply your own favorite tools.

Safety first

Before you begin, make sure you are physically safe. If your teeth and gum symptoms include a fever or difficulty breathing, or you are in unbearable pain that can't be eased, seek out a dentist as soon as possible.

Energetic healing is almost always a slow, sustained process which can be quickly outpaced by serious oral health symptoms. Use metaphysical resources to complement (not replace) necessary dental interventions by easing anxiety, providing clarity, reducing pain and minimizing complications.

As you unpack the energetic or emotional influences on your oral health you may become aware of memories, thoughts or emotions that don't feel safe to explore on your own. If this happens please seek other kinds of support.

That might mean working one-to-one with a therapeutic professional who is sensitive to trauma and nervous system needs, or joining a group program led by a skilled facilitator. It could involve negotiating mutual support with a trusted friend or participating in a peer support group with clear expectations and boundaries. Real support can be found in person, online, on the phone or an app, depending on your preferences, needs and constraints.

Self help

Even if you feel safe, this kind of inner work is often easier when you don't try to do it alone. But when outside support isn't an option, don't be afraid to try working by yourself. This is a golden age for the development and dissemination of metaphysical self-help technology that combines esoteric insights with cutting-edge science of trauma, nervous system support and neuroplasticity.

Science is starting to catch up with indigenous knowledge systems that have linked physical and metaphysical health for generations. There's a growing evidence base for traditional practices and contemporary therapies that are proven to work for emotional and energetic healing. With discernment, some of these therapeutic tools can be easily learned and safe to practice without supervision. YouTube and specialist apps are full of free, helpful introductions to almost every kind of metaphysical self-help modality and there are ever-expanding online courses teaching more advanced applications as well as the basics.

As you explore this book's interpretations relevant to your teeth and gums, you may be overcome with waves of pain, grief, anger, shame or resistance. This process can be a little like giving birth but (unlike labor contractions) you have a choice about when to focus on healing work, so be gentle with the pace you pursue. There's nothing wrong with choosing not to hold space for your hurts when the time isn't right.

Whether you are stepping into this territory alone, or with external support, ensure your body is fed, watered and rested before you try these exercises.

Part of the work can be to ground your insights from these exercises by journaling, as writing and rereading can reduce the need to retrace the same steps of your journey over and over again.

Afterwards, move your body to help release any emotional residue from your system, drink some water (especially if you've had a big cry) and let yourself sleep to integrate any remaining energy.

Anchor in your energetic shifts with consistent practice, healthy habits and embodied action in alignment with your healing intentions. Simple acknowledgment of emotional influences can lead to acceptance or release, transformation or integration. However, the old neural pathways that connect your (conscious or unconscious) memories with your mouth have to be overlaid with new linkages imbued with health and happiness, a process which is reinforced by repetition.

Body awareness

The most fundamental tool in your metaphysical self-help kit is the practice of paying attention to what you feel in your physical body. Use somatic awareness of physical sensations to guide the development of your healing story.

Choose a time when you are safe, rested and undistracted, either supported or in solitude, in a quiet place or out in nature. Start by paying attention to the sensations in your body, without jumping into reaction or interpretation. Explore what emotions, thoughts or images accompany the sensations, welcome those sensations and thank them as allies or messengers.

Allow awareness of uncomfortable sensations or emotions without trying to suppress or escape from them. Notice how they change as your experience unfolds. Resource your nervous system using the techniques described in the following pages to stay present without getting overwhelmed.

Awareness while reading, speaking or thinking

Practice paying attention to what you feel in your mouth as you read the sections of this book which relate to your symptoms, and to the symptomatic parts of your mouth. Slow down as you read. Pause, feel, and think about how my words might apply to your life.

Do you feel:
a chirp of recognition,
the click of a key turning in the lock,
a hazy wall of confusion,
an agitated urge to stop reading/talking/thinking and
do something, anything else than read these words?

Journal on your observations or discuss them out loud with a trusted listener. Continue to notice any physical sensations that arise as you read, think or speak through these ideas. Any of these responses can point to a concept or interpretation that is worth exploring in more depth.

Awareness throughout your day
Check in with your mouth throughout the day whenever you have a quiet moment. Pay attention to your oral posture habits e.g. unconscious mouth movements or positions that you might not notice until someone points them out to you. Any such behaviors could be puzzle pieces that help build out your healing story.

Does your tongue worry at a rough patch
or thrust between your teeth?
Do you gnaw on the inside of your cheek,
suck your lips or blow air behind them?
Do you frequently feel compelled to bite your nails,
chew gum or apply lip balm?
Do you clench and grind your teeth
while asleep or awake?
At what point in your life did the habit start?
Did anyone in your family have a similar habit?
Does the habit remind you of anything?
Does it soothe your uncomfortable emotions?

Aware decision-making
Practice checking in with your body and its inner wisdom when considering any kind of decision, from choosing what to eat to deciding on a new job.

Stop, breathe, close your eyes, and ask yourself
'How does this decision feel in my body?'
Observe:
Where do you feel any kind of sensation?
What is the sensation?
What words could describe it?
If you could see it, what would it look like?

Does it change as you pay attention to it?
Is the sensation a meaningful metaphor
to help you interpret the decision?
For example, does it feel like yes/light/relaxed?
Or does it feel like no/tight/heavy?

Meditation

A regular meditation practice is an invaluable asset for anyone attempting to incorporate metaphysical healing into oral health, both for self-help and as a complementary practitioner or dental professional helping others. Find stillness and create space for inner awareness for at least a few minutes a day.

Focus on your breath.
Pay attention to your physical body.
Notice how the sensations change.
Observe how your experience unfolds.

Supporting your nervous system

Healing physical symptoms happens in both your body and your mind. Emotional hurts and coping patterns that manifest as physical symptoms may require you to bypass your thinking brain and engage directly with your physical body.

The way your brain responds to trauma, and stores it as memories, means that language is limited as a healing resource. In stressful or traumatic circumstances, molecular mechanisms in nerve cells are activated by high frequency brainwaves and receive information about trauma as an electrical charge forming new nerve connections storing vast quantities of mostly *sensory* information about the traumatic experience (Maté).

As you dive deeper into the emotional influences on your teeth and gums you may encounter strong, uncomfortable feelings. Practices such as Havening Techniques or Emotional Freedom Techniques (tapping) can help to soothe your nervous system while releasing or integrating the distressing original underlying sensory information.

Havening Techniques, including self-havening (developed by Dr Steven Ruden, a dentist, and his twin brother Dr Ronald Ruden), can be used with dental phobias, all kinds of troubling memories and mental health symptoms. Havening uses therapeutic touch to change the pathways in the brain linked to emotional distress. The simple safe, self-help technique boosts the production of serotonin in your brain and helps you to relax and detach from upsetting memories or experiences (Youngson).

Emotional Freedom Technique (EFT), aka tapping, was developed by Gary Craig as a way to release emotional blocks by working with the meridian system (Ortner). The technique is simple, tapping your fingers against acupressure points, mostly on your face and upper body. Tapping lightly with your fingers on these spots releases emotional energy. Both Havening and EFT are safe and easy to learn as self-help techniques, with free tutorials available online from many teachers.

You can also support your nervous system with movement, vocalization or breathing whenever you feel resistance, overwhelm or discomfort, especially when you don't have external support available. Practicing nervous system regulation consistently can also be valuable protection by helping build up your emotional resilience so that strong feelings aren't so overwhelming.

Stretching, walking or swimming are some ways to enjoy movement powerfully and pleasurably. You can also try dance, or other expressive movement, to release emotions. Let your intuition guide the kind of movement called in by different feelings. Pay attention to your physical sensations as you move in different ways to express different emotions: wild dancing, slow swaying or curling up tight on the floor then stretching upwards and outwards to take up as much space as possible.

Some expressive movement may come to you spontaneously so

that you notice yourself trembling with fear, shaking with laughter, heaving with tears or stamping with anger. Let these expressions move through you like weather.

When you have strong feelings,
invite the emotion or sensation
to make use of your voice.
Vocalize with moans and whimpers, grunts or groans.
Swear, shout or scream.
Sing, hum, tone or trill.

Deliberately connecting with the Earth in the place where you are right now can help to anchor wild emotional energy. Turn away from the screens that connect you with the rest of the world and be present here and now.

If you can, go outside.
Look around in every direction
and don't take a photo of anything.
Find some ground to sit or lie on.
Take off your shoes.
Push your hands into soil, sand or water.
Plant a seed.
Hug a tree.

Try to eat locally grown food in season, ideally that you have helped to harvest or cook at home. If you are eating out, look for menu items with local provenance. Before eating, pause for a moment of grateful contemplation for how this food connects you more physically to the place where you are right now.

Journaling

Journaling isn't right for everyone, and it's not required for metaphysical healing. However, it can really enhance your healing story's effectiveness, so even if you've never been able to sustain a journaling practice before, it might be worth another attempt to help your teeth and gums.

Journaling is not a substitute for a good therapeutic relationship, but it can make self-help a lot more effective by helping to structure and guide your progress, and making you more aware of the effects of the changes that you're trying. If you are being supported by a therapist, coach or other practitioner, then journaling can make you a more active, self-aware participant in their process and accelerate your progress between sessions.

If you grew up speaking a different language than the one you use now, try journaling in your first language, using the dialect of your childhood and family.

If you are comfortable with visual language, try capturing your insights as doodles, sketches, flow charts or timelines.

There are many ways of journaling, and any of them could be helpful for you. However, there are a few journaling strategies that can elevate any notebook into a healing container: writing by hand, keeping your journal organized, and re-reading what you write.

Write by hand

When you are trying to connect with your inner wisdom, subconscious emotions, childhood memories or ancestral gifts, the tactile experience of moving pen across paper is more likely to get you out of your logical thinking mind. Although capturing notes into your phone can be a great way to collect fleeting thoughts while you are out and about, journaling by hand is a much more connected experience than typing. If you are used to typing for work, study or interactions, then the contrast of handwriting (and its privacy) will help to set journaling apart from your other writing activities.

Organize for reflection

The 'dear diary' stream-of-consciousness type of journaling portrayed in movies or books to surface a character's inner thoughts isn't usually very helpful for healing (at least in my experience). Using a journal to rehearse emotions without resolution is rarely a sufficiently reflective process to develop a healing story. Everyone needs to vent sometimes, but if venting is all you are doing in your journal, then it's not moving you forward.

Take a leaf out of 'bullet journaling' to create a container for reflective writing rather than a continuous day-by-day stream of consciousness. Set up a table of contents on the first (or last) page of your notebook. Number the rest of the pages if needed.

Start a new page (and add it to your table of contents) for each subject or prompt e.g. set up pages for symptom observations or habit tracking by date. Start a separate page for capturing emotional insights about each tooth that needs attention. Whenever you have something new to add on a topic, flip to that page in your notebook and continue writing. If you need more than one page, continue on the next blank page and add its page number to the table of contents.

See the *Appendix of Journaling Prompts* at the end of this book for suggestions of what to write about in your metaphysical oral health journal.

Review and reflect

The single most useful thing you can do with your journal is review what you have written. At the end of a journaling session, scan your day's writing to see what is surprising or especially meaningful. Underline, highlight, or *star* that section; or summarize it with a word, phrase, doodle or sticker.

Every now and then scan your whole journal, letting your eyes catch on the phrases you have marked as most meaningful.

Look for patterns and themes and use those as journal prompts to explore more deeply.

Each time you read your words back pay attention to anywhere you have a strong emotional response. Use those passages as an EFT tapping script, or give yourself Havening touch as you read aloud what you've written.

Developing your healing story

Ask yourself:
What was silent that needs to be spoken?
What was invisible that needs to be seen?
What was denied that needs to be indulged?
What was procrastinated that needs to be practiced?

Your healing story has been living inside your teeth, gums and jaw, trying to make itself known through symptoms. Honest, compassionate self-examination of old hurts and old patterns of coping can help to loosen those stories from where they have been energetically stuck in your mouth.

Identifying and working with your healing story can help you to understand what needs to change for sustainable healing to be possible. Be aware that this process rarely reaches completion quickly. Expect to keep working with it, for weeks, months or even years. Take breaks as needed to resource your nervous system. Capture your story in your journal and/or tell it in therapeutic conversations with a trusted listener so that you can return and reflect on it again and again.

One way to start developing and working with your own healing story is to make note of the messages associated with your symptoms (from Chapter 10) and the archetypes (Chapter 9) and meridians (Chapter 4) located nearest to your symptoms. Then start exploring how these meanings resonate with your life experiences, family history and current circumstances. Expand your interpretations from what is currently snagging your attention, to see how your symptoms fit into the bigger picture of your life.

Looking at the big picture may bring uncomfortable memories back into your awareness or stir up difficult emotions but working with a healing story doesn't require you to revisit every excruciating detail. You don't need to relive every trauma you have survived. Rather it can be sufficient to identify the broad patterns and themes that have reappeared throughout your life. Healing comes as you give space to the emotions and sensations that arise as you play with your insights, rather than from poking old wounds until they bleed.

Take on the roles of a researcher of your circumstances, a historian of your life and an analyst of your environment. Be willing to courageously dig deep into your story. Your teeth are energetic storehouses, and your symptoms are asking for you to clean out the energy that doesn't serve you or the planet, from your own experience and your family lineage.

Pay attention in granular detail to what you feel and think when you touch your jaw or mouth. Embrace love, forgiveness, gratitude, compassion, generosity and humble 'beginner's mind' towards your oral health. If you feel anger, frustration, self-loathing, shame, fear or grief, try to observe those feelings with relaxed curiosity to understand the part those emotions play in your healing story.

Here are four possible ways to develop and work with a healing story: by creating a map or a timeline, by identifying what needs to change in your life right now and by retelling your story in different ways.

Visual mapping

Draw a base map of your own mouth. Use it to document the dental treatments you can remember. Identify the parts of your mouth that have been asking for attention through symptoms at different times. Mark where you've had teeth filled, crowned, pulled, capped or aligned. Note any baby teeth that stayed past the usual age, or any adult teeth that never grew in. It may be helpful to look through any information that you've received from dentists, or if necessary, ask your current dentist to email your notes or last treatment plan.

Then create metaphysical maps that overlay your base map based on interpretations of your unique combination of symptoms, archetypes and meridians provided in Part II of this book.

Dental timeline

Create or talk through a dental experience timeline. If you're journaling, and especially if you've had a lot of dental treatment, try the following approach:

- For a lifelong dental history write a column of numbers representing the years of your life from birth until now down the center of a double spread in your journal (using as many pages as needed). If your dental problems are new, make the timeline start about one year before you first became aware of symptoms.
- On the left page, note whatever you remember of your dental history at each age including symptoms, treatments, orthodontia etc. Enhance your timeline with colors, doodles, arrows, dotted lines of connection, or whatever you want to make it richer and more meaningful for you.
- On the right page, note what was happening in your life around the time of each dental experience. Include your state of general health, mental health, significant relationships including family, friends and romance, stressors from study or work, moving house, other big events or significant travels.
- Note any medications, recreational drugs or health-impacting habits including dietary experiments, exercise programs or mindfulness practices.

- You may find it helpful to check old calendars and dental receipts or talk to family members to help you fill in more details about your dental and life timeline.

On subsequent pages of your journal (or in therapeutic conversations) you can start to cross reference your timeline with the map of metaphysical associations suggested above. Open yourself up with relaxed curiosity to new, perhaps unexpected, insights.

What needs to change now

Sometimes a healing story will point you towards an aspect of your current life that isn't supporting your highest good. Looking at your current circumstances can be the easiest place to start making sense of the messages from your mouth, especially with the recent onset of an acute issue.

One of the roles played by your teeth and gums is to let you know when you should stop settling for less than nourishing food, jaw-tightening stress levels or carelessly harmful hygiene habits. Unhealed emotional trauma responses can be the reason you don't give your mouth sufficient physical support to be healthy.

Your symptoms might make sense when your daily activities are not in alignment with your soul purpose or you feel stuck. Your teeth and gums thrive best when what you do from day to day supports your values, enables growth and learning and moves you towards your goals and dreams.

Your mouth can be sensitive to how well you feel seen, heard and loved. Try thinking about your symptoms in the context of your relationships right now, rather than as a completely individual experience. Gums may be more resilient when your boundaries are clear to you and clearly communicated to others. Your teeth might be reacting to a difficult breakup or struggling with the hard work of staying together through challenges or vulnerable in the transition into a new stage of family life with children arriving or leaving.

Retell your story

Sometimes it can take weeks of chewing on these ideas before you get clarity. You won't always recognize your story right away. Sometimes you will think – not this old trauma, surely my twenty years of therapy and healing must have resolved this by now. Or maybe you will think – that's too trivial, I don't have enough emotional attachment for this to explain my symptoms. But there is no experience or insight that is too trivial, too obvious or too familiar to be part of a healing story.

Keep brainstorming metaphors and experimenting with associations. Don't be afraid to extend your pool of possible healing stories by drawing on memories, dreams, insights from other people, or even song lyrics that catch your ear.

Use imagination, metaphors and cultural references that resonate for you to tell your story. I have worked with clients who incorporated their God, goddesses, angels, dragons, animals, aliens or fairies as allies in their healing story. We've worked with inner children, ancestors, past lives and lost twins. We've visited imaginary beaches, travelled to other planets, dropped into other centuries or traversed across millennia.

See also, *Tell your own healing story (and hold it lightly)* in Chapter 3.

INNER CHILD OR INNER INFANT

When first I met Eve in her sixties, she described her mouth as 'the ruins of a besieged city'. Although talented, educated and creative, she also felt ashamed to smile or speak in a way that showed her missing teeth. She was sick and tired of pain in her mouth, and she felt scared and hopelessness about her future oral health. She was single, living alone in the South-Western United States, working remotely in a new job and struggling with basic self-care such as healthy eating and oral hygiene.

Eve was born with a cleft lip and a cleft palate. Her mother had responded to her newborn baby with fear and guilt, while her father expressed revulsion and shame. Baby Eve couldn't breast-feed, and even had trouble bottle-feeding until her first surgery on the cleft when she was two weeks old. Her family tried to keep her hidden until she had a second surgery at two years old which closed the cleft. She never grew tooth 9, the Nurturer archetype.

By the time we started working together, every tooth in her top jaw was filled, crowned, capped or missing. When Eve was sixteen, orthodontists had broken her jaw 'for realignment'. By middle age, she had no molars left after multiple root canals failed and were extracted. The only intact teeth in her mouth were her bottom incisors, the archetypes of Guardian, Beast, Doll and Martyr.

Eve described her past dentists and oral surgeons as sadists and herself as having dental phobia. Even though she couldn't remember her first experience with surgery in her mouth at two weeks old, every dental experience since had been affected by that original trauma. Her adult experiences of social isolation and haphazard self-care had been imprinted in her infancy when she learned to believe that she was unworthy of care and attention.

Painful, powerless or scary experiences in your infancy or childhood can get stuck in your brain, so that you respond to situations in your adult life like a scared, powerless child. The inner child is not so much a memory as a trauma response or survival pattern. Whatever age you were at the time of a traumatic experience is probably the age of your inner child, and you may have many inner children who are trying to keep you safe because they represent parts of you that are still living in your past.

Working with your inner child can sometimes feel like hostage negotiations, as though this part of you is still experiencing a dysfunctional, traumatic childhood. Inner child work can be hard because overwhelm and confusion feel like present time (even though it's all old stuff).

Soothing your inner infant

The younger the age of the inner child who needs attention, the less effective language and logic are as healing strategies. Eve spent months nurturing her inner infant – specifically that part of her nervous system which was still feeling everything as she had as a newborn. Eve's painful front teeth (around the cleft scar) still held the energy of a baby who was wild with hunger for food and touch, while frozen in the horror of her parent's reactions to her.

We found that her inner infant wouldn't respond to words but could be soothed with loving touch. Eve used Havening Techniques to self-soothe her inner infant by stroking her palms together, brushing her hands along the outsides of her arms from shoulder to elbow, and caressing the curve of her cheek and jaw where nerve endings are particularly sensitive to a mother's comforting touch. Gradually Eve's relationship with her top teeth began to shift from oppressive pain to empowered partnership.

Another way to soothe an inner infant is to hum like a mama comforting her beloved child. The vibrations from humming can be particularly soothing for traumas trapped in gums or jawbone.

Sometimes an inner infant crying for attention through your teeth just needs to know they are loved and cared for. You can use a small object like a smooth crystal or tiny soft toy to represent your tooth/inner infant. Keep this avatar with you all day (in a pocket, tucked into your bra over your heart, or nestled under your pillow) so that your tooth is constantly reminded that it is cared for and loved.

Speaking the language of your inner child

Helen came to see me because she was struggling with chronic problems affecting the roots of her lower right molars (archetypes: Rival, Professional and Goals). Helen's immigrant parents speak a Chinese dialect that Helen describes as very harsh and direct especially between adults, without any way to express sadness and lacking nuances of softness and wistfulness. She and her older brother were born in the United States but Helen's parents switched from using baby talk to severe adult tones when she was only five, so their words have always sounded critical and disappointed to her ears.

Helen's first root canal happened while she was studying for medical school entrance exams, which she ultimately didn't sit. When we met she was trying to avoid another root canal while she and her new (Italian-American) husband were living with her parents. The young couple were searching for a home of their own nearby while Helen started up her Chinese folk medicine practice.

For many of my clients who are bi- or multi-lingual immigrants or children of immigrants, language appears to play an important role in understanding and healing their oral health issues. This can also be a factor for anyone who learned to 'code switch' between the way their family spoke in the home and the dominant version of the same language used at school, on media and in the workplace.

Try using the language, dialect or accent that was your first language, or the language of your parents, when you are working on adverse childhood events, family patterns or intergenerational traumas. If you feel ambivalent or uncomfortable with the way adults speak your first language, try incorporating a little baby talk into your healing story, while paying close attention to your physical and emotional responses.

Play with your inner child

Dominic was first diagnosed with gingivitis when he was only nineteen, which advanced to periodontitis despite regular deep cleaning and vigilant self-care. By his late thirties, several teeth felt loose in his eroded jawbone. He anxiously and obsessively checked the black spaces appearing between his teeth where the gum was diminishing. When his plans for significant gum surgery were interrupted by the Covid-19 lockdowns, Dominic started searching for a metaphysical approach to gum healing.

Dominic uses Internal Family Systems Therapy, studies meditation and facilitates men's groups. He is a devoted father and emotionally articulate husband. Nonetheless, he felt intensely anxious about his periodontist's grim prognosis when he found me.

He had already done much of the dark difficult work of healing a traumatic childhood. More and more of our work together started to focus on embracing pleasure, play and joyful self-expression to help his gums to thrive. Embracing these healing qualities had to be balanced by attending to worries about not being seen as a serious adult man.

As Dominic paid attention to these aspects of himself that felt anxious, sad or ashamed, he could identify his inner child at different ages with emotional hurts from those times. He pictured what each inner child was wearing and the environment they appeared in to gain clues about how to try and meet needs that the inner child wasn't able to articulate.

One definition of trauma is having no control in a scary situation, so play can be a low-risk way to help your inner child to heal feelings of powerlessness. Everyone has different ways they can enjoy playfulness to release trauma from their body.

Play is also a way to integrate your inner child into your adult life so that they can experience and enjoy the power and autonomy of being a grownup, instead of staying stuck in your powerless past. Play enables you to access the gifts of your inner child; the innocence, creativity, awe, delight and freedom that you were born with. Take all the time you need to create feelings of safety as you keep checking in with your inner child so that they can notice it's safe to relax and have fun in your life now.

The more connected your inner child is with your adult life, the more they will be able to believe that the lack of safety and control of your childhood is in the past not the present. Bring your inner child into your daily life to share fun and make (age-appropriate) choices, e.g. allow your inner child to choose something you will wear today, even if it's only a silly undergarment.

If you have young children around, try bringing your inner child out to play with your real children. Remember how you liked playing at the same age as your offspring or young friend. Invite your inner child to engage with blocks, dolls or video games with all the curiosity, imagination and presence of your younger self.

Ancestors

Alongside the inner children stuck in your teeth and gums, there may also be an accumulation of ancestral trauma. Past generations' experiences of collective trauma from war, famine, slavery, forced migration, oppressive gender roles or religious/racial persecution can etch oral health vulnerability into DNA and family culture, to be expressed as teeth and gum issues in later generations.

In Dominic's family, such traumas had been passed down through generations of dysfunctional fathers and sons, until Dominic encountered his destiny as the cycle breaker. As a sensitive and spiritual young man he came of age at the turn of this century in a cultural milieu starting to challenge notions of gender, masculinity and whiteness. But without being acknowledged, the family's historical traumas became embodied in his gums.

Eduardo Duran writes that trauma is not only passed on intergenerationally, it is also cumulative (quoted in Hübl). When trauma isn't dealt with in the previous generation, subsequent generations have to deal with it.

Dominic had spent his adult life working full time in the family's manufacturing business where his almost-eighty-year-old father was still very much in charge. Dominic's inflamed gums embodied both his frustration with his father's lack of emotion and attachment to power; and grief for his beloved uncle (the only adult who seemed to have time for young Dominic) who had died the year before his gum issues started.

Include your ancestors in your healing story

Dominic developed a powerful, imaginative, healing story tracing his way back over generations of disconnection from the Divine Masculine. Knowing his ancestors had lived in Northern Italy, but that his surname was Huguenot, we speculated that his paternal family lineage had experienced forced migration in the seventeenth century to escape religious persecution and massacres in France.

Forced off lands where they had lived for centuries, the Huguenots lost their history, their livelihood and their indigenous connection to place. Dominic's ancestors became unwilling immigrants, first to Italy where the Huguenot diaspora jostled uncomfortably alongside a resentful local population, then to a North America where colonizers had already displaced the original inhabitants and the myth of meritocracy ultimately favored white men.

As with many white family histories, Dominic's ancestors experienced both ends of each axis of oppression, prejudice, and economic inequality. One stressor that is common to both victim and oppressor identities is a disconnection from one's full humanity, which can be particularly harsh for people who feel like their survival depends on performing extreme masculinity. In patriarchal societies, any expression of emotions (other than anger) can threaten their tenuous place in the power hierarchy, and so grief, loneliness or shame get suppressed, to become embodied into the physical DNA and cultural norms inherited by subsequent generations.

Stories get hidden from view because people don't want to feel the pain of remembering. But the hurt didn't disappear when the stories stopped being told or the emotions stopped being expressed.

The emotions attached to these stories get stuck in your body.

Attend to your nervous system, to the somatic experiences of being in your body as you learn and retell these stories, and regulate your nervous systems as you do so. Observe the prickling tears, the churning stomach or the tight jaw and breathe into that part of your body. Rather than pushing through the feelings, make sure you stop to cry, nap or move.

Dominic was so hurt by the way his father abused his role as the family patriarch that he had rejected ever being in such a role himself. For Dominic, ancestral healing also meant finding and practicing positive forms of masculinity by clarifying and reinforcing healthy boundaries. He needed to allow feelings of discomfort as he inherited the mantle of patriarch at work and in his family and chose to wear it with emotional intelligence.

Researching and retelling your foremothers and forefathers' lives as healing stories may help to release their trauma and secrets from the dark recesses of your mouth. This process of remembering can be a powerful way to support your descendants, both biological and any younger people whose lives you may influence. Working to heal your oral health issues can be a catalyst for breaking family cycles of trauma response.

When I caught up with Dominic recently, he reported that his gum symptoms were much stabilized and his father was spontaneously acknowledging Dominic's leadership for the first time.

Honoring your ancestors

When you honor your ancestors they can stop clamoring for your attention with distressing teeth and gum symptoms. In some families it may seem like the totality of the legacy is their suffering and strife embodied into your mouth as disease. Ancestral healing works best when you can honor your ancestors without lingering in their pain.

Sometimes honoring ancestors may seem wrong because you feel critical or ashamed of your family history. If that's how you feel, try to seek out more information, or use your imagination to give context to the individuals and their actions. Every ancestor lived a life that included more than their experiences as victims or oppressors. They were complex, unique human beings with the strength to survive long enough to bring another generation into being and that strength has continued through the generations to you, even if it was buried in sorrow or shame.

Your ancestors can be a loving, supportive presence in your healing. Open yourself up to receive the gifts of your ancestors – their strength, intelligence, determination, or sense of connection that enabled them to survive the trauma that you inherited.

Research your family history and and/or your cultural heritage. Ask elders to share their memories, do genealogical research or read relevant history books. Connect with benign contemporary celebrations of your cultural or religious heritage.

Share any known ancestral and family stories with children to help bring legacy and continuity into their conscious understanding for future generations. Use your imagination and intuition to explore possible histories or alternate histories, or to allow your ancestors' voices to speak into your journal, or be heard in a therapeutic conversation.

If it feels appropriate, when pictures of your parents, grandparents and great grandparents are available, place these where you can see them often. Consider decorating the space around these images with special mementos or fresh flowers. You could light a candle or incense nearby. When you look at your ancestor's picture, you can say a prayer, ask them questions, or tell them about your day.

THE TIP OF THE ICEBERG

The self-help tools in this chapter are just a taste of the many possible ways to work with the metaphysical associations of your oral health issues. If you practice meditation, try to meditate on your healing story. If you do therapy, talk about messages from your mouth with your therapist. Many energetic modalities can be focused on your mouth to good effect.

At any point, if you get stuck or feel lost in the process, turn back to the Manifesto in Chapter 3 to situate yourself within the guard rails I've recommended. And remember, this work is intended to be complementary, so if your symptoms get worse instead of better, please see a dentist. Sometimes a dental intervention is necessary, even when there is a strong metaphysical influence.

12.

HEALING WITH GRACE

Viola could smell the infection festering inside a gum pocket on her lower right, so deep and with bone loss so severe, that the first molar was bifurcated, exposing the gap between roots. Viola couldn't see, but could imagine, the exposed roots standing up from her jawbone, separated like flower stalks appearing too delicate to hold up the weight of their big back molar. But she needed that tooth to continue to act as an anchor for one of the bridges replacing adult teeth that had never appeared, even after her retained baby teeth were extracted as a young adult.

At the age of 67 Viola's mouth was a patchwork of gold and porcelain: fillings, caps, crowns and bridges. Tooth 30 was her last remaining first molar on that side, since the opposing upper tooth was extracted. She came to me determined to do everything in her power to save her remaining teeth and heal her gums. Her healing journey had taken her to a series of six different dentists, each contributing a piece to the holistic healing puzzle.

Through a process of contemplative and energetic inquiry and dialogue with her tooth 30, the name Grace had come to Viola. She felt, processed, and released deep guilt about decisions she made to extract her mother's teeth (when her mom Lucy was suffering with dementia). In a self-forgiveness process, her mother came through as St. Lucia, pouring white healing light into the top of Viola's head. Stuck emotion melted into kindness and empowerment.

The Tooth Archetypes described in Chapter 9 can be thought of as job descriptions. They sum up generic, idealized roles that your actual teeth may embody most fully when they experience symptoms. The way each tooth fulfills its archetypal role is unique to you. You may visualize your tooth 30 (Professional) as a graceful saint, or an aspiring circus performer. You may imagine your tooth 3 (Name) as a past life warrior or a beloved grandfather.

Intellectually interpreting the metaphysical messages of your mouth won't heal symptoms. Your symptoms don't only embody childhood struggles, family secrets or ancestral traumas, just as your oral health is not only influenced by your diet, hygiene habits and jaw tension.

Your teeth and gums also cry out for you to be true to yourself right now. Your teeth really want you to be living a good life as an individual and in relationships. Your teeth want you to feel happiness, pleasure, and fulfillment. This might be hard to believe when your teeth are giving you trouble, but they only hurt when you are not in alignment with whatever a good life really means for you.

Viola stayed exceptionally consistent to a complex protocol of herbs, homeopathic remedies, supplements, and mindful cleaning rituals for many months. She spent 45 minutes every day on meditation, breathing and sound healing exercises. She spoke directly with Grace and the rest of her oral community including 'Jack' (once tooth 3, now a tender loose area of gum under a Nesbit partial bridge), 'Ruby Rose' (the gingiva) and 'Ruth' (the alveolar part of her jawbone). Working in concert with the many strong entities that she imagined occupying her mouth, immersing herself in their stories and trusting the intelligence of the whole system, she allowed her inner world to be a catalyst for change in her outer life.

Over the years I have noticed that the people who have the worst chronic problems with teeth and gums – those of us who have more fillings than enamel, multiple root canals or multiple lost teeth, or severe chronic gum disease – tend to take *everything* seriously. We share a feeling that life is quite hard, we have to struggle, and that we don't deserve for things to be easy.

As a coach I've also observed that the people who get the best results from using holistic teeth healing strategies – those who are actually able to successfully prevent root canals, remineralize cavities or restore their gums – are those most willing to embrace living with more joy and more pleasure, with a sense of fulfilling their soul purpose in a light-hearted and playful way.

Grace's lingering soreness ceased around the same time that Viola felt she could no longer visualize conversations with her. When her dentist said that tooth 30 was dead, with no more heroic measures possible to save it, Viola told me 'I feel that Grace had a hospice passing – going in her own time and her own way. I think that's the shift that happened when I was no longer feeling her presence.'

After working to heal her gums for seven years, Viola finally felt ready to have the tooth pulled to make way for a new, comfortable, good-looking bridge across the back of her lower right gums.

As she meditated with her teeth prior to the dental visit, she felt the energy of dancing and clicking of heels. She heard 'a way will be revealed by group intuitive intelligence'.

When she met with the dentist and his team, they had changed their minds about their treatment plan and were curious to see how long tooth 30 might be able to last with a rare procedure to amputate only the root with the most infection. An innovative solution had appeared, and the procedure unfolded seamlessly.

Different parts of your mouth are aligned with different aspects of the truth of your essential goodness, the gifts of your ancestors and the highest potential of your humanity. Tooth decay, gum disease and other symptoms can be understood as alarms calling your attention to stuck energy that's getting in the way of the full power and possibility of your soul essence. Symptoms exist to prompt you to heal the blocked emotions that obscure your true self.

Viola's spontaneous identification of the community of characters occupying her mouth opened the door for me to develop the thirty-two Tooth Archetypes at the heart of this book. My system of Tooth Archetypes is indebted in no small part to the gracious way Viola shared the secret lives of her teeth and gums.

CONTINUE GROWING, DEVELOPING AND LEARNING

If you have the kind of teeth or gums that always have a lot to say, by which I mean you have had chronic oral health problems, then listening to the messages in your mouth is probably going to be a lifelong practice. There will always be more to learn from, and about, your teeth and gums. However, by being sensitive and responsive to their messages when they are most subtle can help to ensure that symptoms don't escalate and lead to irreversible damage.

Understanding and working with their metaphysical meanings is valuable because it can enable physical support strategies including dental procedures to work more effectively and sustainably. Your teeth and gums have been trying to take care of you for your whole life. They've been holding onto suppressed emotions so that you could survive, to function, to do as well as you have done, despite all the hard things you have been through. Now it's your conscious mind's turn to take responsibility.

*Make time to listen to your teeth regularly
with relaxed curiosity.
Follow their cues and lean into learning
and experimenting as you respond.
Show your mouth appreciation with pleasurable
flavors and sensations,
mindful hygiene, laughter and song.
Lavish your teeth and gums with love, attention,
gratitude and forgiveness.
You are the boss of your mouth, so be a good boss.*

APPENDIX OF JOURNALING PROMPTS

SOMATIC SYNONYMS

Tune in to your awareness of your symptoms: their sensations, emotions, effects, appearance etc. Write a list of words that describe your symptoms, e.g. blocking or eroding or aggravating, deep or shallow, nagging, intermittent, subtle, overwhelming, irritating, invasive, unbalanced, stuck etc. It can be helpful to refer to a thesaurus or do a synonym search to help you find more descriptive words.

Once you've written down at least six words that describe your symptoms, cross reference them with the pages in Part II that are relevant for your mouth, to help you identify non-symptom experiences your descriptive words could apply to as metaphors. Write a sentence or more about each word on your list, leaving a space between each sentence to add notes later.

For example: you are preoccupied with a toothache in tooth 13 and your list of descriptive words include *deep, overwhelming, persistent, throbbing* and *nagging*.

It's on the left, so you might write about something in your personal life that feels *overwhelming*.

It's on the upper jaw, so you might write about a *deep* desire that remains unfulfilled.

It's adjacent to the lung and large intestine meridians, so you might write about *persistent* grief.

It's a second premolar, so you might write about how often you *nag* your children.

It's the Harvest archetype, so you might write about a *throbbing* sense of deprivation.

Extra credit: After a day or two, reread what you have written, and note any common themes or linkages. Could these sentences be rearranged to tell a story?

INTERVIEW WITH AN ARCHETYPE

Write down a conversation between you and the tooth archetype that you want to understand better, as though you are writing a script. This is easiest to do if you meditate for a few minutes, creating a calm, peaceful, compassionate space inside yourself and then invite the archetype to meet you there. Welcome it with compassion and gratitude. Then open your eyes, pick up your pen and start by writing a question such as 'how are you?', 'what's going on?' or 'what would you like me to know, do or change right now?'.

You can do this with the archetype for any tooth including one that is missing or root-canaled. I recently journaled a conversation with my tooth 7, the Inner Critic archetype, the site of my first root canal when I was a mortifyingly self-critical seventeen-year-old. There's nothing wrong with the tooth now, but because I was feeling very self-critical I decided to meet with the archetype.

I asked the tooth archetype what it wanted me to know, and it filled half a journal page with all my self-critical anxiety about this book and everything else going on at the time. Then I imagined bathing the tooth in love until my Inner Critic giggled and squirmed in response. Sense of humor restored, I continued journaling a conversation that went something like this:

Me: Hey, you know I want to share my book with as many readers as possible because I can imagine so many ways it will improve people's lives.

IC: But you've been devastated in the past by grand ambitions that led to disappointment and shame; I don't want you to suffer like that again.

Me: Thanks, I know... Hey, you really got stuck in that homeless-unemployed-dropout mess when I was 17 didn't you?

IC: That was a bad time. I don't want that again.

Me: Me either. But you know I'm a grown-up now.

IC: But it's so scary and so many things could still go wrong because you are so disorganized, unprepared and unprofessional.

Me: I'm sorry you feel so scared, but it's OK, I'm organized enough and actually it's okay for me to make mistakes and not be perfect.

IC: Noooooooooo! (little tantrum)

Me: You're very cute.

IC: What? I'm root canaled and I broke and then the crown kept breaking until you got the short crown and now I make you lisp.

Me: I know, you're adorable, and I'm so grateful you're still a presence in my mouth all these years later.

IC: Well...OK. I mean I do my best and I only want what's best for you.

Me: I know. Thank you. Hey, did you know, you are in my book?

IC: Me? You think I'm that important?

Me: Oh sweetheart, you are front and center in my life always.

Extra credit: Transcribe a conversation between more than one of your tooth archetypes. What do they have to say to each other? How do they interact?

PLOT POINTS AND CHARACTER STUDIES
- Write about the relevant associations in Part II as though you are writing a book report for a novel you've read, or you're making notes about a novel that you are going to author.
- Write about your symptoms' messages as plot points that unpack the characters of the tooth archetypes and tooth types that apply to you.
- Give your tooth archetype characters the emotions associated with their adjacent mouth meridians.

FAMILY HISTORY
- Write down what you know, or can find out, or can imagine, about your parents and grandparents' life stories, especially those elements that resonate with your metaphysical mouth map.
- Write a (factual or imaginary) history about your more distant ancestors and cultural heritage that is cross-referenced with your metaphysical mouth map.
- Write a letter to a parent, grandparent or distant ancestor about your life and/or your oral health. Ask them for help or advice. Let them know if you are hurt or disappointed by them. Thank them for anything you appreciate about their legacy, inspiration or the gifts you inherited.

WRITE A LETTER
- Dear [symptom] I want you to be healed because… and this is how I think it can be done…
- Dear [tooth archetype], I appreciate your… I want to release your…
- Dear [extracted or root-canaled tooth], I'm sorry you…
- Dear [inner child], thank you for figuring out how to survive… Let me tell you about how good things are now that I'm grown up…

- Dear tooth, I want you to know…
- Dear tooth, secretly I wish…

Extra credit: How does it feel to write such such a letter?

INTENTIONS, PLANS AND PROBLEMS SOLVING

- Write about what you want to heal or improve in your mouth.
- Write about how it will feel to have your oral health problems fully resolved: in your mouth? In the rest of your body? In your day-to-day life? In your relationships? In your work?
- Do you believe it's possible to achieve that outcome? Why or why not?
- What do you think you might have to change to achieve that outcome? With your nutrition? With your hygiene? With your general health? With your community? With your relationship to dentists? Which of these changes are within your circle of influence?
- What is the most loving and compassionate way to move towards healing?
- Describe an imaginary celebration meal with friends, family, or a date, once your oral health issues are fully resolved. Imagine what it is like to smile widely, laugh uninhibitedly, speak freely and eat and drink whatever you want without a care.
- Write a list of affirmations for your teeth and gums. A) State the healthy outcome you want for your oral health with positive emotions in the present tense: e.g. I enjoy flashing my bright white toothy smile. B) Describe the active process of healing with positive emotions: e.g. I delight in supporting my gums with daily flossing.
- Brainstorm everything you could do in response to the messages you found through metaphysical mouth mapping.
- Write down three baby steps you could take this week.

- Write a list of the best things to do when your symptoms are active.
- Write a list of good things to do when you feel anxious about your oral health symptoms.
- What do your teeth and/or gums need from you this week?
- What seems to be the biggest obstacle to healing? Brainstorm five possible ways to handle it differently.
- How can you make more space in your life for healing?

Visual journaling prompts

- Draw an outline of the shape of the tooth you want to heal, then draw, paint or collage inside with colors or images that represent the tooth's meanings for you, or which represent that healing.
- Draw an outline of the shape of the tooth you want to heal, and outside the line draw, write or collage words and phrases describing what you want to release, ease, exclude or heal (e.g. pain, hardship, loneliness etc.). Inside the line draw, write or collage the qualities you want to create, attract and embrace (e.g. calm, love, abundance etc.).
- Draw, paint or collage a portrait of your tooth archetype.
- Download free full-size, quick-reference PDF charts for locating tooth archetypes and mouth meridians from www.holistictoothfairy.com/charts

REFERENCES

BOOKS

Beyer, Dr Christian, *La nueva interpretación de la caries: Los orígenes psicoemocionales a través de la decodificación dental* (Spanish edition, translated by Gloria Roset Arisso), El Grano de Mostaza Ediciones (2016).

Caffin, Dr Michèle, *Quand les dents dévoilent le mystère de l'homme de A à Z*, (French edition), Guy Trédaniel (2015).

Clarke, Arthur C, *Profiles of the Future: An Inquiry into the Limits of the Possible*, Bantam (1962).

Hay, Louise, *You can Heal your Life*, Hay House (1984).

Hübl, Thomas et al, *Healing Collective Trauma: A process for integrating our intergenerational and cultural wounds*, Sounds True (2020).

Jung, CG, *C.G. Jung Letters*, volume 1, Adler G and Jaffé, A (eds), translated by RFC Hull, Princeton University Press (1992).

Maté, Gabor, *When the Body Says No: The cost of hidden stress*, Scribe (2003).

Menakem, Resmaa, *My Grandmother's Hands: Racialized Trauma and the Pathway to Mending our Hearts and Bodies*, Central Recovery Press (2017).

Ortner, Nick, *The Tapping Solution: A revolutionary system for stress-free living*, Hay House (2017).

Rose, Evette, *Metaphysical Anatomy: Your body is talking, are you listening?* volume one, version 2.8, Evette Rose (2012).

Schwartz, Richard, *No Bad Parts: Healing trauma and restoring wholeness with the internal family systems model*, Sounds True (2021).

Segal, Inna, *The Secret Language of Your Body: The essential guide to health and wellness*, Beyond Words (2010).

Van der Kolk, Bessel, *The Body Keeps the Score: Mind, brain and body in the transformation of trauma*, Penguin (2014).

Youngson, Robin, *Time to Heal: Better me, Better world*, Rebel Heart (2020).

Articles

Akcali, A et al, 'Periodontal diseases and stress: A brief review', *Journal of Oral Rehabilitation*, 40, no. 1 (2013).

Arnold et al, 'Medicine's inconvenient truth: The placebo and nocebo effect' *Intern Med J.* 44(4) (2014).

McDermott, CL et al, 'Early life stress is associated with earlier emergence of permanent molars', *Proceedings of the National Academy of Sciences*, 118 (24) (2021).

Chu, Courtney, 'From personal to popular: The Westernization of traditional Chinese medicine', coldteacollective.com (2020).

Costa, Dora L et al, 'Intergenerational Transmission of Paternal Trauma among US Civil War Ex-POWs, *Proceedings of the National Academy of Sciences*, 115, no. 44 (October 30, 2018).

Folayan, Morenike Oluwatoyin, et al, 'Association between adverse childhood experiences, bullying, self-esteem, resilience, social support, caries and oral hygiene in children and adolescents in sub-urban Nigeria', *BMC Oral Health* 20, no. 1 (July 11, 2020).

Ford, Kat et al, 'Understanding the association between self-reported poor oral health and exposure to adverse childhood experiences: A retrospective study', *BMC Oral Health* 20, no. 1 (February 14, 2020).

Gleditsch, J, 'Oral acupuncture', musculoskeletalkey.com/oral-acupuncture (2016).

Kirkengen, Anna Luise and Lygre, Henning, 'Exploring the relationship between childhood adversity and oral health: An anecdotal approach and integrative view', *Med Hypotheses*,m 85(2) (August 2015).

Knoblauch, Uta et al, 'The association between socioeconomic status, psychopathological symptom burden in mothers, and early childhood caries of their children', *PloS One*, 14, no. 10 (2019).

Marchant, Jo, 'Placebos: Honest fakery', *Nature*, 535 (2016).

Orr, Sara and Lovatos, Amber, 'The Impact of Adverse Childhood Experiences on Oral Health', *Registered Dental Hygienists* (July 15, 2021).

Qi X, et al, 'Social isolation, loneliness and accelerated tooth loss among Chinese older adults: A longitudinal study', *Community Dent Oral Epidemiol* (January 17, 2022).

INDEX

A

Abandoned, 83, 101, 110, 113, 116, 119

Abscess, 9, 20, 30, 125–126, 137, 142

Acupuncture, 52–53, 55

   Acupressure, 55, 153

   EFT, 55, 153, 157

   Reflexology, 52, 55

Adult teeth, 9, 27–28, 68, 71–72, 137, 139, 159, 171

Affirmations, 180

Alveolar bone, 33, 35, 133–134, 136

Ancestors, 16, 19–20, 28, 135, 141, 143, 161, 166–169, 174, 179

Anger, 45–46, 53, 61, 88, 126, 129, 149, 154, 158, 167

Ankylosed teeth, 9, 126–127, 137–138

Anxiety, 5, 7, 17, 20, 40, 45, 60, 62, 123, 141, 148, 177

Apex surface, 83

Astrology, 42, 57, 71–73, 75–77, 80

Authenticity, 52, 65, 78, 101, 120

Authority figure, 87, 91, 96–97

B

Baby teeth
  Retained, 9, 138–139, 159, 171
  Timing, 27–28, 72–73
Bacteria, 26–28, 32–33, 35, 56, 79, 132, 134, 142–143
Beyer, Christian, Dr, 9, 28–29, 56, 67, 73, 77, 81–83, 94–95, 114–115
Blood, 31–34, 113, 122, 126, 130, 140
Body dysmorphia, 85, 90
Bone loss, 9, 35, 39, 133–134, 136–137, 171
Boundaries, 70, 87, 92, 94, 103, 132, 134, 136, 148, 160, 168
Braces, 54, 75, 126, 137
Brain, 26, 29, 31, 34, 42, 152–153, 163
  Brain development, 28, 56, 74
Breathing, 13, 16, 25, 118, 120, 125, 127, 148, 151–153, 168, 172
Bridge, 137–138, 171–173
Broken teeth, 9, 129–131, 144
Bruxism, 9, 34, 127–130, 133, 137, 140
  Clenching teeth, 44–45, 127–130, 151
Buccal surface, 81–82

C

Caffin, Michele, Dr, 9, 56–57, 71–77, 80
Calcium, 31–32, 34, 54, 76
Canine teeth, 9–10, 27, 60, 73, 95–99
Canker sores, 9, 130, 137
Caries, 9, 83, 131–132
Cavitation, 39, 126, 138
Cavities, 7, 9–10, 56, 79, 81–82, 123, 131–132, 142, 144, 173
Cementum, 33, 133, 136
Cervical surface, 82
Childhood, 16, 102, 110, 123, 129, 135, 139, 155, 162, 164–165, 171, 186

Children, 44, 49, 53, 65, 76–77, 98, 100, 105, 114, 121, 142, 144, 160–162, 166, 169, 177

Chipped teeth, 9, 128, 132, 144

Circadian rhythms, 54

Colonialism, 44, 85, 90–91, 119

Community, 8, 48, 65–66, 97, 117–118, 129, 135, 137, 172, 174, 180

Competition, 18, 66, 107

Cracked teeth, 9, 128–131, 140, 143–144

Creativity, 65, 73, 75, 98, 105, 135, 155, 161, 165

Crowns, 30, 54, 137, 171

Cynicism, 62

D

Decay, 9, 33, 79, 81–83, 95, 114–115, 123, 131–133, 142–143, 174

Deciduous teeth, 11, 28, 139

Demineralization, 34, 130, 132, 140, 143

Dental chart, 10, 51, 56

Dental interventions, 14, 17, 25, 30, 37, 39, 54–55, 123–124, 137, 148, 170

Dental timeline, 159

Dentin, 31–32, 54, 132, 140

Dentinal flow, 31–34, 54

  Parotid gland, 23, 32–33

Dentists, 5, 10, 14–15, 44, 81, 127–128, 134, 137, 140, 159, 162, 171, 173, 180

Dentures, 54, 137–138

Depression, 14, 61, 107, 118

Distal surface, 82

DNA, 19, 27, 69, 121, 166–167

Dreams

  Aspirational, 64–65, 110, 115, 160–161

  Sleep, 42, 110, 138, 161

Dry mouth, 35, 133

E

Emotional freedom techniques (EFT), 55, 152–153, 157

Energy healing, 23, 47

Exploitation, 89, 95, 98, 118–119

F

Family, 89, 96, 98
  Family history, 16, 21, 42, 139, 158, 166–169, 179
  Family of origin, 66, 85, 93, 114
Father, 69, 71, 86
  Father figure, 29, 69, 101, 109–111, 114
  Paternal, 22, 27, 114, 119, 135, 167
Fear, 17, 20, 30, 35, 45–46, 53, 60, 62, 116, 118–119, 127–128, 134, 138, 154, 162

Femininity, 69, 71, 89, 108–109

Fertility, 85, 100, 112

Fever, 125, 148

Fillings, 14, 30, 39, 48, 171, 173

Frenula (central), 60

Front teeth, 11–12, 26, 29–30, 35, 60, 65, 68, 70–71, 81, 83, 163

G

Gaslighting, 103, 120–121

Gender, 17, 44, 69, 85, 92, 109–112, 119, 166

Gingiva, 33, 133, 135, 172

Gingivitis, 9, 39, 122, 133, 135, 164

Gum conditions, 9, 126–127, 133–134, 138, 144
  Bleeding gums, 122
  Gum Recession, 10, 133–134, 142–143
  Gum Tissues, 33, 133–134

H

Havening, 152–153, 157, 163
Healing story, 21, 41–44, 150–151, 156–158, 160–161, 163, 167, 170
Herbs, 7, 22, 172
Homophobia, 19, 85, 115, 119, 137
Hygiene, 7, 14, 90–91, 118, 121, 160–161, 170, 175, 180

I

Immigration, 14, 90, 109, 141, 166–167
Implant, 30, 39, 54, 137–138
Incisors, 9, 27, 60, 68–72, 84–94, 162
Infection, 7, 9, 20, 30, 35, 39, 55, 79, 125–126, 131, 133, 137, 140, 171, 174
Inner child, 161–166, 179
Intuition, 22, 64–65, 85, 104, 110, 121, 153, 169

J

Jaw, 7, 13, 15, 23, 27, 30–34, 45–46, 62, 64–65, 67, 73, 127–128, 138–140, 157–158, 162–164
  Jaw clenching, 44, 127, 160, 168, 172
  Jaw clicking, 128
Journaling, 10, 149–150, 154–160, 169, 176, 181
Jung, Carl, 138

K

Kabbalah, 57
  Hebrew letters, 71–73, 75–77, 80

L

Labial surfaces, 81
Language, 8, 18, 25, 40, 73, 77–78, 89–90, 112, 118, 136, 152, 155, 163–164
Left side of mouth, 11–12, 64–65, 67, 69
Lingual surfaces, 81–83
Loose teeth, 125, 128, 133–134, 136–137, 139

Lymph, 33, 126

M

Magnesium, 31–32, 80
Masculinity, 69, 71, 110, 166–168
Meditation, 42, 47, 98, 120, 152, 165, 170, 172
Meridians, 7, 51–55, 58–63, 177, 179
Mesial surfaces, 82
Metaphysical influences (vs physical), 17, 123–125
Missing teeth, 5, 9, 137–139, 142, 161, 177
Molars, 9, 12, 21, 27, 35, 61–62, 66–67, 76–78, 108–117, 162–163
Mother, 27–29, 45–46, 69, 86, 115–116
  Maternal, 27, 46, 100, 109, 113, 117, 121
  Mother figure, 69–70, 85, 90, 100, 108, 113
Mouth breathing, 25, 127
Mouthguards, 54, 128

N

Nagging, 53, 176
Nerves, 23, 31, 33–34, 54, 140
  Nervous system, 14, 127, 148, 150, 152–153, 157, 163, 167–168

O

Occlusal surface, 83
Oral microbiome, 7, 25–28, 34, 123, 142
Oral posture, 7, 123, 127, 151
Orthodontia, 54–55, 75, 154, 159
  Orthodontists, 68, 75, 137, 162

P

Pain, 5, 13–15, 20, 25–26, 31, 36, 40, 45–46, 69, 123, 125, 129, 131, 140, 143, 148–149, 161, 163, 167–168
Parents, 14–16, 22, 28–29, 66, 69, 71–72, 76–77, 100, 110, 136, 143, 163–164, 169

Patriarchy, 87
Periodontitis, 9, 133, 136, 164
Permanent teeth, 11, 27, 137, 139
Physical influences (vs metaphysical), 17, 26, 123–125
Piercing, 16, 54
Plaque, 9, 32, 35, 137, 142–143
Premolar teeth, 9, 11–12, 20, 27, 61–62, 73–76, 99–108, 137
Pulp, 31–34, 54, 56, 140

R

Racism, 19, 85, 115, 119, 137
Rejection
  Rejection of implants, 39
  Social rejection, 62, 100, 114, 121
Religion, 22, 62, 66, 117–120, 160, 167, 169
Resistance, 44–46, 139, 149, 153–154
Right side of the mouth, 11–12, 65, 69
Root canal, 13–15, 20–21, 23, 30, 39, 137, 162, 164, 173, 177

S

Safety, 34, 60, 76, 90, 92–93, 101, 165
Saliva, 31–32, 34–35
Secrets, 5, 17, 82, 114, 168, 172, 174
Self-help tools, 148–150, 152, 170
Sensitive teeth, 9, 34, 37–38, 122, 128, 131, 133–134, 137, 143–144
Sexism, 19, 115, 119, 137
Sexual abuse, 29
Sexual pleasure, 103
Sexuality, 44, 69, 85, 109–111, 121, 135
Shame, 5, 43–46, 60, 76, 85–86, 91–92, 112, 114, 118, 121, 135, 149, 158, 161–162, 165, 167, 169, 178
Silence, 82, 86, 93, 109
Silent treatment, 89, 103, 106

Slavery, 19, 95–96, 99, 166

Somatic awareness, 24, 36, 38, 86, 90, 126, 150, 168, 176

Speaking, 6, 25, 33–34, 55, 73, 89–91, 96–97, 100, 107, 118, 129, 150, 155, 163–164

Stress, 8, 17, 21, 29, 32–35, 48, 54, 77, 127–133, 135, 141, 144, 152, 160, 167

Suppressed emotions, 18, 61, 88, 125–127, 167, 174

Swollen gums, 37, 125

Symptoms
  Acute, 135–136, 160
  Chronic, 15, 21, 136, 138, 163, 173–174
  Mild, 39, 48, 133, 135, 143
  Symmetrical, 67

T

Tartar, 9, 32, 133, 137, 142–143

Throbbing, 13, 125, 140, 176–177S

TMJ disorder, 129

TMJ, Temporomandibular joint, 9, 62, 127–129

Tongue, 26, 30, 35, 37, 52–53, 55, 82, 130–131, 151

Tooth enamel, 54, 128, 132, 142, 144

Tooth extraction, 29–30, 54, 75, 137–138, 162, 171–173, 179

Traditional Chinese medicine (TCM), 8, 46, 52–53, 58–63

U

Ulcers, 9, 130

W

Wisdom teeth, 9, 11–12, 27, 46, 59, 62, 66, 73–74, 77–80, 117–121, 13

ACKNOWLEDGEMENTS

First and foremost, I offer thanks to all my Holistic Tooth Fairy coaching clients who were willing, and often eager, to work with the emotional and energetic influences on their particular oral health issues. Our deep and sustained explorations of their childhoods, family histories and recent circumstances in relationship to their symptoms taught me more about the metaphysical meanings of teeth and gums than any other source.

I'm especially grateful to the small subset of clients who agreed to let me write about them (anonymously) in this book; sometimes patiently working through several iterations of their story to find a version that remained true to their experience while also aligning with my didactic aspirations.

Thanks to the diverse folks on the Insight Timer meditation app who share their dental worries in my regular 'Messages from your Mouth' sessions. Your questions on our live video sessions allowed me to refine my intuitive interpretations into robust concepts and language that resonate across cultures and generations.

Acknowledgements

Writing a book, although a solitary endeavor, couldn't happen without many people's encouragement, support and help. Thank you to Conrad Johnson, my writing accountability buddy, for our weekly phone calls (and cat videos); Philippa Jamieson for editing; Martin O'Connor for proofreading; Amanda Sutcliffe for design; Élisabeth Denis and Adot Studios for helping with some of the illustrations; Amanda Collins for helping with translation (and cheerleading); Danny for sharing his research into metaphysical aspects of gum health; Meredith and Dr Robin Youngson for reading, self-publishing advice and hosting LOLW as an early focus group for me; Sarah Chann, Megan McLean, Anna Rajan and Joy Love for reading early versions, Michelle Whitehead for co-working and sound advice; Eleanor LeFever for always believing in me; Fatin Zainudin and Zoë Taylor for keeping the business side of the Holistic Tooth Fairy ticking along when my attention was elsewhere; Donna Powers for services to video and games; Larnie Bell for our many conversations about the impacts of colonialism and racism on oral health; and last but not least thanks go to my family especially my daughter Louise, my mother Martha, and my late father, Norman, who passed away while I was still writing this book.

Special thanks to my mentors: Pip Kempthorpe (Business Mentors New Zealand) who got me started; Andrea Schroeder's Dream Book coaching and Impossible Dream journals which kept me going; and Monica Leonelle and Russell Nohelty's Kickstarter Accelerator which helped me finish. And speaking of Kickstarter, thank you to the 160+ backers who believed in my work enough to pre-order *The Secret Lives of Teeth*.

Enduring gratitude goes to my three-legged feline soulmate, Phryne, who was invariably distracting, unhelpful and often downright obstructive to the writing process (believing that there's nowhere better to sit than a keyboard that's in useeeeeeee) and yet she kept me feeling cozy and loved throughout.

ABOUT THE AUTHOR

Meliors Simms (she/her) is the Holistic Tooth Fairy, a natural oral health coach who has worked with hundreds of clients all over the world to avoid unnecessary dental procedures and have better experiences with the necessary ones. After a diverse career (from policy research to craft arts) and a lifetime of terrible teeth troubles, she stumbled on an alt oral approach which prevented what would have been her seventh root canal. That inspired years of independent research and experimentation, eventually leading to her uniquely holistic approach, the Holistic Tooth Fairy Way. Learn more about the Holistic Tooth Fairy Way at holistictoothfairy.com

Made in United States
North Haven, CT
01 March 2024